PRAISE FOR *WELCOME TO THE JUNGLE*

"Hilary Smith brings to light what those with bipolar already know: that just because you've been diagnosed with a mental illness doesn't mean you've lost your insight, intelligence, or playful (and often self-mocking) sense of humor. *Welcome to the Jungle* astutely captures the roller coaster of emotions that accompany bipolar— from trenchant despair to uproarious mania— and does so in a way that never alienates the reader, but rather sucks you in and keeps you wanting to go along for the ride. Writing with a wisdom and faculty well beyond her years, Smith had me laughing out loud—not at her, but with her. Whether you're a teen for whom the diagnosis of bipolar is as raw and fresh as a snipped nerve, or in your twenties struggling with the disease for what seems like decades, *Welcome to the Jungle* is the quintessential young person's companion."

—Malina Saval, author of *The Secret Lives of Boys: Inside the Raw Emotional World of Male Teens*

"Hilary Smith's wise, hilarious, and candid book is a veritable lifesaver not only for those suffering from bipolar disorder, but for those struggling to keep their sanity while loving them. Maybe because the author suffers from the disorder herself, her book is an actual survival guide, brimming with insight, anecdote, and tough love. Recovery was never so inspiring."

—Allison Burnett, author of *Undiscovered Gyrl*

D0005573

"By far the best, most comprehensive self-help book out there about bipolar disorder. Hilary Smith's incredible sense of humor, candor, and wit make her guide easy to read, a pleasure, and a laugh riot. Every person with bipolar (or family member or friend) should read this book as soon as possible. This book will save lives."

—Andy Behrman, author of *Electroboy: A Memoir of Mania*

"Funny, smart, and unflinchingly astute, *Welcome to the Jungle* is exactly the guide you want on your journey from chaos to stability as you learn to manage bipolar disorder. Smith's sure voice is a welcome companion over some hard road, and her wry wisdom lights the way. Indispensable."

—Marya Hornbacher, author of *Madness: A Bipolar Life* and *Wasted: A Memoir of Anorexia and Bulimia*

HILARY SMITH

WELCOME TO THE JUNGLE

EVERYTHING YOU EVER WANTED TO KNOW ABOUT **BIPOLAR** BUT WERE TOO FREAKED OUT TO ASK

Conari Press

First published in 2010 by
Red Wheel/Weiser, LLC
With offices at:
500 Third Street, Suite 230
San Francisco, CA 94107
www.redwheelweiser.com

Library of Congress Cataloging-in-Publication Data
Smith, Hilary, 1986–
Welcome to the jungle : everything you ever wanted to know about bipolar
but were too freaked out to ask / Hilary Smith.
   p. cm.
ISBN 978-1-57324-472-5 (alk. paper)
1. Depression in adolescence—Popular works. 2. Manic-depressive illness
in adolescence—Popular works. 3. Smith, Hilary, 1986—Health. 4.
Manic-depressive illness in adolescence—Patients—Canada—Biography. I.
Title.
RJ506.D4S585 2010
616.85'2700835—dc22

                   2009050798

Cover design by Sara Gillingham
Text design by Donna Linden
Typeset in Perpetua and Toronto Gothic

Printed in Canada
TCP
10 9 8 7 6 5 4 3 2 1
The paper used in this publication meets the minimum requirements of the
American National Standard for Information Sciences—Permanence of Paper
for Printed Library Materials Z39.48-1992 (R1997).

CONTENTS

INTRODUCTION

This is a book about bipolar disorder. Or if you're a free spirit or an R. D. Laing enthusiast who doesn't believe in a pathological explanation of your extreme mood states, it's a book about living with the highs and lows everyone *else* in North America is calling "bipolar disorder" (the punks!). I'm supposed to use this introduction to tell you my personal story about being bipolar, but that can wait.

Right now I've got a hankering to write about shin splints.

I got shin splints when I was thirteen. They hurt. My Anglophilic boarding school made everyone participate in enforced jaunty after-school sports (and, every spring, supposedly jaunty sniper drills on the lawn). After a single week on the cross-country running team, jogging along behind the meaty-calved senior boys, my shins started to feel weird. Little shoots of pain sprang up each time my shoes hit the pavement. It really hurt, but I winced and kept running. If I ignored the problem, it would probably fix itself. Four practices went by. I limped along. During the fifth practice the coach (of whom I was terrified) rode up behind me on a bicycle and shouted, "Stop running! You're limping! Go to the infirmary!"

Confused and embarrassed, but relieved, I turned around and walked to the school physiotherapist's office, where a team of smokin' hot sports therapists treated me for shin splints. Going to physio was fun and cool: there were always tons of people there getting their ankles wrapped or their sprains ultrasounded, or just hanging out in the whirlpool drinking from sketchy-looking Nalgene bottles. The physiotherapists teased me about letting my shin splints get so bad without asking for help. I did the stretches and exercises, got a better pair of running shoes, and eventually started running again.

Total days of pain: less than five.

Social approval of shin splints: high.

Overall experience with shin-splints diagnosis and treatment: supercool!

Six years later, I was a junior at the University of British Columbia, majoring in English literature. No more sports, no more sniper drills. This was the West Coast, baby—poetry readings, pot, and rainy-night house parties. I lived in a funky old house in Kitsilano that had a rich history of student debauchery and was known to several generations of UBC students as the place to go for anything involving mint juleps and knife throwing. Six of us lived there, and it got *loud*.

In January of that year, I started having trouble sleeping. Writing it off to the constant noise and stimulation in the house, I didn't pay much attention. By February I couldn't sleep at all, and my mind was swimming in thoughts and rhymes. Box! Fox! Haha!

In lectures, I either scribbled furiously in the diary I carried with me everywhere, recording my urgent insights ("He was an ornithologist. He was bornithologist into it!"), or I stood up abruptly to leave partway through and weep in the bathroom or wander in the forest that surrounded the campus. At parties, I would give my phone number to several different guys, then panic and jog home through the night, all the way from East Van to Kitsilano. At my part-time job as a bagel-stand cashier, I would prop my ever-present diary over the cash register and worry about the people who came to buy bagels: whether they knew what I was thinking, if they might be interested in coming to a fabulous party I was planning. At night, I would lie down in bed as a formality, then spring back up ten minutes later when sleeping didn't work out. Eventually, the mental chatter in my mind intensified so much that it felt like there were "four of me" whose constant arguments and repartees were alternatingly sinister and hilarious.

It really hurt, but I winced and kept going. If I ignored it, it would probably fix itself. Time passed. I limped along. Even though whatever was wrong with me was more pronounced than a physical limp and should have been more obvious, there was no coach to ride past on a bicycle and shout, "Stop running!"

So I didn't.

I felt like a ceiling light whose switch was stuck in the on position. Whatever I did, I couldn't turn myself off. Confused and tormented by my condition, I nevertheless strode through the days, handing in essays, going on dates, and calling my parents long distance for normal, how's-the-weather conversations. Even though I was falling apart inside my head, I wasn't *doing* anything that had enough obvious craziness to attract anyone's attention. Not running down the street in my underwear. Not trying to convince the bank teller I was Jesus. Just wandering around having thoughts that went off like sparklers and a body that had forgotten how to fall asleep.

When I finally went to see a doctor at the walk-in clinic down the street, it wasn't because I wanted to help myself or because I thought I might have a medical disorder. It was out of shame. I had started crying and rambling in front of my roommates one night because I couldn't sleep, and I felt so embarrassed for crying in front of them that I was determined to get sleeping pills so it wouldn't happen again. I waited in the exam room, feeling guilty for taking up the doctor's time when there were three-year-olds with runny noses waiting to be seen, and when the doctor came in, I started crying all over again. When she asked what was wrong, I blurted, "I can't do this anymore!"

That's when someone finally said, "Stop running."

Over the next few weeks, I went through the usual mental-illness maze of being misdiagnosed with unipolar depression, becoming hypomanic (again) from antidepressants, being rediagnosed with bipolar II, and choking down a series of different antipsychotics and mood stabilizers until I hit on a combination that didn't make me want to bury myself in a hole. I spent a lot of time in the waiting room of the UBC hospital, which was neither fun nor cool, because everyone there either had an STD or a mental illness and there was no freaking whirlpool.

Total days of pain: lots and lots.

Social approval of bipolar: not obvious.

Overall experience with bipolar diagnosis: kinda really bad.

My dad flew out from Ontario to see how I was doing and make sure I wasn't completely crazy. We blasted through the Chapters bookstore in downtown Vancouver, and he bought me every bipolar-related book on the shelf. We made a stop at the Starbucks. As we were power walking down the street, my dad hailed a taxi midsentence, hopped in, and rushed off to catch his flight back to Ontario. I stood on the sidewalk with a bag of bipolar books in one hand and a half-finished Green Tea Frappucino in the other.

The party was just getting started.

In the days that followed, I returned most of the bipolar books and used the money to buy poetry books—not because I wasn't interested in the former, but because they made me feel tainted and messed up. They were too adult, too clinical, too alarmist, clearly written for family and caretakers at their wits' end, and designed to look authoritative and medical. They didn't answer any of the questions I had about bipolar, and I felt like a huge tool for even having them in my room, their ALL CAPS titles blaring out at the world. I thought there should be a book that was a little more honest, a little more badass, and a little more sympathetic to the average teen or twenty-something's first experience of the mental-health system.

So here's that book.

This book is mainly about how to live with bipolar, but it's also about how to *think* about bipolar. Sure, you can think of bipolar as a chemical imbalance in your brain, but you can also imagine it as a video game, a shamanic journey, a crash course in existentialism, or a plain old pain in the ass.

If you're reading this book and you've just been diagnosed with bipolar disorder: welcome to the jungle. Hope you brought bug spray, 'cause the spiders in here are as big as your face. Taken your meds? Good.

Now let's get started.

1

WHAT JUST HAPPENED?
LIFE BEYOND THE DIAGNOSIS

How did it happen?

Maybe you were doing a research project on the Beatles, and by the end of the term you thought you were one of the Beatles. Maybe you were trying to find a girlfriend, and at the end of a futile year of looking you were trying to die. Maybe you were having a perfectly happy summer that turned into an ecstatic summer or a winter sadness that never lifted when spring came. The sun was shining, cars were honking, the radio was playing something catchy. You were toasting a bagel, playing Xbox, talking to your best friend about the afterlife, or tuning your guitar.

Then the mothership landed.

You were diagnosed with bipolar disorder. This big whale of a diagnosis slid over the sun, and your world was suddenly held hostage. A hatch slid open and out came doctors, psychiatrists, pills, hospitals, and self-help books. They strapped you to a gurney and scrawled "bipolar" on your chest in permanent marker. "I'm not bipolar!" you shouted, struggling in your restraints. "She's bipolar! He's bipolar! Anyone but me!" They gave you two Depakote and a glass of water. "Misdiagnosed!" you snarled, gulping it down.

Eventually, the mothership flew away, but left its cargo behind. Medication, doctors, and bipolar were here to stay. You picked your way out of the rubble, the last one standing after an earth-shattering encounter. You're alive, but now you have bipolar. Your ray gun is strapped to your side; your freshly acquired jar of anti-psychotics and mood stabilizers is on your other hip. You step out of the doctor's office.

WHAT JUST HAPPENED?

Dealing with a bipolar diagnosis can be just as hard as the unfettered depressive or manic episodes that led up to it. It's like you've been hit by a truck, only to be told at the scene of the accident that you're going to be hit by several more trucks of steadily increasing size over the course of your life (have fun with that). For a while, it's hard to think about anything else but the fact that you're screwy enough to be considered mentally ill, and especially hard to accept a diagnosis of mental illness if you've always considered yourself a happy, healthy person. The diagnosis looms over your life, and you just want to rewind to a time before it happened. *Can anything be the same again? How did they even decide I was bipolar?*

Being told you have a serious mental illness is a co-lossal mind fuck. What does "bipolar" even mean? And what does it really say about who you are? This chapter is about understanding what the people in white coats were thinking when they made the diagnosis. Even if you hate everything to do with jargon and psychiatry and labels like "bipolar," you should know this stuff so you understand what (and who) you're dealing with—because, after all, there's a good chance you are going to be dealing with it for the rest of your life.

BIPOLAR? SAYS WHO?

Your doctor didn't just look at you and decide you had a bipolar face. Unfortunately, there's no blood test for bipolar disorder, but there are fairly rigorous guides in place to reduce the odds of being misdiagnosed (though people get misdiagnosed all the time). Doctors try to avoid a misdiagnosis by ruling out all the other possible causes of your symptoms before making a diagnosis of bipolar.

There are four things a psychiatrist takes into account before making a diagnosis of bipolar disorder: your current symptoms, your medical history, your family history, and your psychiatric history. Doctors see hundreds and hundreds of people and know what to look for. They look for patterns ("Wow, that guy talks in a constant stream without any pauses, and he hasn't slept for a week. And his uncle is bipolar, and he's taken four jobs") that are consistent with bipolar. You, of course, are a beautiful and unique snowflake, but like it or not, there are a number of classic behaviors and indicators (big and small) that people experiencing mania, hypomania, or depression in our culture tend to present. Quibble over details all you like, but if the shoe fits in five places, they're sticking that sucker on your foot. P.S. Hope you like Velcro.

THINGS THAT GO INTO A BIPOLAR DIAGNOSIS

1. CURRENT SYMPTOMS

Do you *seem* depressed or manic? Have you mentioned being unable to sleep, unable to think straight, or crying all the time? Are you talking fast? Of course, *you* may feel that you are acting normally, but it's very hard to reflect accurately on yourself. Over time, a psychiatrist will be able to compare your "manic" or "depressed" behaviors to your "baseline." (For example, the psychiatrist might figure out that you just *always* talk fast. It's just who you are, no big deal.) But for a first diagnosis, the only thing they can really compare you to is the general population.

2. MEDICAL HISTORY

Do you have another disease, like epilepsy or diabetes, that might be causing your symptoms? Are you on crack? Pregnant? Have a brain tumor? Or are you just hungry? Many medical conditions share symptoms with bipolar. You want to rule these out as possible causes before deciding the diagnosis is bipolar.

3. FAMILY HISTORY

It's taken as a given that your uncle Bernie is off his rocker, but has anyone else in your family been diagnosed with a mental illness? Have any of your relatives been hospitalized for depression, mania, or psychosis? Anyone receiving counseling or taking meds for a psychiatric disorder? Bipolar has a strong genetic component, and bipolar in the family can predict bipolar in you.

4. PSYCHIATRIC HISTORY

Did you get diagnosed with unipolar depression three months ago, and now you have so much energy you can't sleep? Have you ever been diagnosed with another psychiatric disorder? The doctor will want to rule out unipolar depression, schizophrenia, and other possible psychiatric causes for your symptoms. The doctor might ask you to draw a "mood chart" of the past twelve months or several years. (I know, he's lame, but he can probably help nonetheless.)

"BIPOLAR" IS A WORD FOR A PATTERN

You didn't get diagnosed with bipolar because you're ugly or because the doctor doesn't like you. Let's face it—he's uglier, and his personality needs improving. You got diagnosed bipolar because your symptoms more or less fall into a common, distinct pattern, observed in millions of people. We're currently calling that pattern "bipolar" and treating it with pharmaceuticals and talk therapy. In the past, the same pattern has been called by a different name (hello, "hysteria") and treated by different means (like lots of cold showers). In the future, it will undoubtedly be called something else entirely and treated with mind melding and cosmic nanoprobes. In other cultures, what we call "bipolar" has other names and other symptoms and explanations entirely.

Psychiatric illnesses aren't like herpes. You can say, "You have a cold sore, therefore you have oral herpes," but you can't say, "You have insomnia, therefore you are bipolar." Insomnia can be explained by a hundred different reasons; cold sores are always due to herpes.

A bipolar diagnosis doesn't extract something hidden in you and reveal it ("All along she was a mutant!"); it merely describes what's already there ("Ah, these symptoms are part of the bipolar pattern."). Being diagnosed bipolar doesn't change you and make you into something you weren't before; it just says, "Hey, you're a person who could probably benefit from taking mood stabilizers!"

Thinking of your diagnosis this way is much less painful than thinking of it as a life sentence or a siege on your identity. No matter what the psychiatric community wants to call it, you're still you—whether you have bipolar, hysteria, a wandering womb, or just plain sand madness. Everybody else changes their mind about what to call it, so there's no reason why you can't too. Don't think "bipolar" is an accurate description of your experience? How about Chronic Sleep Taxationitis or Acute Porn Star Overidentification Syndrome? No matter what you call it, no matter how you think about it, no matter how you treat it, you're a person—not a collection of symptoms or an entry in the *DSM-IV* (the hefty diagnostic manual produced by the American Psychiatric Association that you've probably seen lurking under your psychiatrist's desk). Nothing can change that. Don't dwell on whether or not "bipolar" is the perfect way of describing your condition; just consider whether the solutions available for bipolar are helpful for you.

DEALING WITH THE DX

Being diagnosed with bipolar disorder is akin to waking up after a wild night of intoxication to discover that at some point during your (fuzzily remembered) antics, you went and got a tattoo on your bicep. Not just any tattoo—you got a big old snake-eating-a-unicorn tattoo. That sucker's six inches high and three across. It's kind of badass, kind of hideous. You stare at it in shock. You vaguely remember going to the tattoo parlor, *but why?!* You frantically think back to the chain of events that might have led up to you getting a tattoo of a snake eating a unicorn. You feel guilt, anger, embarrassment, denial, nausea—the whole ride. Eventually you realize you're going to have to live with this thing for the rest of your life, and from here on, your attitude towards your new tat is entirely up to you.

WORDS, WORDS, WORDS

The field of psychology has words for everything. It has a word for when you talk too fast. A word for when you talk too slow. A word for when you smear your feces around your bedroom.

It even has a word for your reaction to being diagnosed. Reject the diagnosis? You're "underidentifying" with being bipolar. Want to make sweet love to it? You're "overidentifying" with your bipolar characteristics ("Ha ha, that was just soooo bipolar of me"). The endless labeling is alienating, but since you're going to run into it, you might as well be prepared.

THE SNAKE-EATING-A-UNICORN GUIDE
TO OVER- AND UNDERIDENTIFICATION

So you wake up with this tattoo/diagnosis. How do you react?

Underindentification: "Ho ho ho! This is surely but an amusing temporary tattoo placed on me as a prank. It will certainly wash off in the shower."

Medium-Low: "The tat is real, but I'm going to wear long-sleeved shirts for the rest of my life to cover it up."

Middle: "Living with this tattoo is going to be a bitch and a half, but it's also kind of dope."

Medium-High: "Short sleeves for me, baby."

Overidentification: "This tattoo defines me, man. I'm going to tattoo the rest of my body with snakeskin and have a horn surgically implanted on my head."

THE NON-METAPHORICAL GUIDE TO OVER- AND UNDERIDENTIFICATION

When you underidentify with your diagnosis, you reject it and don't want to integrate it into your identity. You might think there's been a mistake. Or you might accept that you have a disorder called "bipolar," but don't want it mentioned ever again.

When you overidentify, you attribute too much of your identity to bipolar disorder. Maybe you go over your past with a fine-toothed comb, ferreting out clues that everything you've ever done was a result of having bipolar genes. Or you drop all your other activities and spend all your time on bipolar message boards, interpreting everything anyone says in terms of GABA receptors.

Many people experience the full spectrum of under- and overidentification over the course of the first year, or several years, of being diagnosed with bipolar disorder. One day you accept you're bipolar, the next day you weep bitterly over it, the next day you don't even think about it. Even though I was diagnosed with bipolar disorder several years ago, there are still mornings when I wake up and say, "Really? *Really?*" Then my boyfriend rolls over and says, "Really." And I say, "Oh, yeah."

LET'S TALK ABOUT FEELINGS

However you're feeling about your diagnosis, there's someone out there feeling the same way. There's another newly bipolar skater punk grieving over her "lost self," another type-A personality feeling guilty for "screwing it all up," and another nerd who's done his research (helloo, Medline) and who feels that in his professional opinion, the doctors are right, but more research needs to be done in the area of gabapentan interceptors. You might even have every one of these feelings at different points throughout the year and throughout your life:

"There's no way this can be true."

"Finally, an explanation!"

"This is a mistake."

"This is my fault."

"This is so cool."

"It's my parents' fault!"

"I should have been stronger/smarter/more careful."

"This makes sense."

"I can't believe this is happening."

"Is my life ruined?"

"Can I still graduate/be a poet/find a boyfriend/have a career?"

"Am I going to die?"

"I wish I could turn back time."

"I shouldn't have dropped so much acid."

"I shouldn't have left the church."

"This feels like a dream."

"This is completely ridiculous."

"I can't tell anyone."

"Bipolar's for pussies. Real men/women don't have bipolar."

"Bipolar's not a real disorder. Psychiatry is a conspiracy."

"What the hell?"

"Scientology! Kaiieee! Kaieeee! Take me, Lord Xenu, I'm a level one clear!"

"I guess the only thing I can do with my life is become a belligerent hobo."

"I was already a belligerent hobo."

"What am I going to do with my life?"

"I can't live with this."

"Why didn't someone tell me sooner?"

"Will people just shut up about this?"

"Am I going to be on meds my whole life?"

"Does this mean I'm crazy?"

"This is unbearable."

"This doesn't really make a difference."

"So what?"

"What a blessing!"

You're going to go through long stretches of your life when the fact that you have bipolar disorder never crosses your mind—and there will also be the odd stretch when you can think of nothing else. Trust me: you'll get used to it.

WHY DO I HAVE BIPOLAR?

You didn't get bipolar because you're weak, lazy, bad, or because Zeus wanted to smite you (though a meditation instructor I talked to claimed bipolar was due to bad karma from a previous life; people, don't step on ants!).

You probably got bipolar because you were genetically predisposed to it, and something triggered those particular genes to light up howling. The triggering of that genetic time bomb is called "onset." The age of onset for bipolar disorder is generally between the late teens and late thirties, though nowadays kids and old people are getting diagnosed too.

If you're feeling guilty about developing bipolar, don't: there's really nothing you could have done to avoid getting it, short of strangling yourself in the womb. Some people who have the genetic potential never develop bipolar (just like you can have a family history of breast cancer without developing it yourself). If the sucker happens to break out, well then, you did nothing to cause it except simply be alive.

People who have bipolar always have a certain narrative about how it developed: "I'd just gotten my first job and my first girlfriend, my parents divorced, and I started going crazy." "I was staying up late, listening to a lot of Marilyn Manson, and shit just started getting weirder and weirder." For one thing, humans love to tell stories. It makes much more sense to place bipolar disorder in the context of certain events, rather than having it come out of nowhere. Though the environmental triggers of bipolar disorder are not well understood, one thing many accounts have in common is a period of lifestyle change, stress, or major life events (both positive and negative). Real specific, huh? Try naming a time in your teens and twenties when you're *not* going through a period of stress, lifestyle change, or major life events!

In other cultures, narratives of mental illness sometimes focus on spiritual matters ("he is being haunted by ghosts!") or family relations rather than biochemistry. Our Western narrative might be scientifically accurate, but it is not necessarily the most useful or compassionate way of imagining mental illness. If "haunted by ghosts" feels more meaningful and accurate to you than "haunted by misbehaving neurotransmitters," then please, tell your own story!

Otherwise, it's you against the mothership. Lock and load, lock and load. . . .

PROGNOSTICATING (E.G., "AM I SCREWED FOR LIFE?")

I get a Google news feed about bipolar disorder: any news article with the word "bipolar" gets sent to my inbox. Every day I get several police reports about missing persons who are "diagnosed with bipolar disorder and thought to be off their meds," as well as a rash of news pieces about murders and suicides involving people with bipolar disorder. Now look me in the eye. Do you have bipolar? Yes? Are you, personally, going to become a missing person or a murderer? Probably not. There are things in life you can control and things you can't, but if you get your act together as much as possible, given your personal circumstances, and do it *early*, then your chances of having a wonderful, happy, interesting, completely Google-news-feed-unworthy life are great.

While everyone's prognosis is different, it generally boils down to this: if you have bipolar disorder, your life is going to include some periods of crushing depression, some periods of whacked-out mania or hypomania, a whole lot of meds, perhaps a psychotic episode here and there, and maybe a hospitalization or two (or ten). You can experience all those things and still have a fun, meaningful, productive life.

Look at it this way: you're building a cabin in the woods, but a hurricane comes through and when it's over all you have is a few measly planks of wood, a saw, and some nails. Do you set the wood on fire, step on the nails, saw off your legs and cry about it, or do you chop yourself some new wood, build yourself a cabin, and have a great life? Everything is up to you. You have exactly the same power over your destiny as you did before you had bipolar—now you're just working with a different set of materials.

All you have are the fabulous resources of your own mind to realize your potential. Bipolar or not, you still have choices to make, and you're the only one who's going to be making them.

EIGHT WAYS TO PROVE YOU'RE NOT BIPOLAR

1. Keep a straight face and neutral affect at all times. This will demonstrate how completely stable your mood is.

2. Whenever you hear something about bipolar disorder on the news, laugh loudly and say, "Ho, ho, ho, I'm so perfectly twitterpated to not be affected by such a foreign and fearsome affliction as that!"

3. Paint rabbit faces on your meds so they look like recreational drugs. Wear furry clothing and plastic beads so people think you're a raver.

4. When you get hospitalized, tell everyone you know you're an "investigative journalist" doing an exposé of what it's "really like" to be hospitalized.

5. Hire a look-alike to impersonate you at social events when you're too depressed to go out.

6. Surround yourself with people who are more extreme than you (drama students, nonrecovering addicts, circus people). In contrast, you will look totally un-bipolar.

7. Start a fake blog about your completely normal, nonbipolar life. Include entries such as, "Fun day at the mall!" and "New kitty is cute!"

8. Get a high-powered career that could never be held by a person with a mental illness. That will show them!

2

MANIA, DEPRESSION, PSYCHOSIS, OH MY! A WHIRLWIND TOUR THROUGH THE EPISODES OF BIPOLAR DISORDER

Sometimes, crazy people have crazy emotions. A lot of the time, crazy people have completely normal emotions. This section discusses the technical definitions of mania, depression, psychosis, rapid cycling, and mixed states, and also discusses what they aren't. After all, it's crazy to attribute all your emotions to having bipolar.

I'M NOT MANIC, I'M JUST HYPHY

Before we get into all this bipolar stuff, let's talk about hyphy. Hyphy is a Bay Area hip-hop style characterized by people dancing or acting in a hyperactive, ridiculous manner. You put on your stunna shades, get blasted, and "go stupid." One particularly prestigious way of "going stupid" is to put your car in neutral and dance on the hood while it rolls forward without a driver; this is called ghost-riding the whip. E-40 and Mistah F.A.B. wrote entire songs about ghostin'.

Now, when you think about it, all this going stupid sounds a lot like a manic episode: substance abuse, hyperactive speech and dancing, risky and grandiose activity—feelin' like a star. Yet thousands of otherwise sane, asymptomatic ballers get hyphy every day, and nobody accuses them of having bipolar disorder. What's the difference between being manic and plain old gettin' hyphy?

MISTAH F.A.B.'S GUIDE TO THE *DSM-IV*

Hyphy	"Dude, Bro, let's ghost-ride your car then put it on YouTube, Bro, ha ha ha. Babes will dig it. Wooooo!"
Hypomanic	"Dude, bro, stop the car, we're going to ghost-ride the whip right-now. Yeah yeah, stop the car. We need to do it right now right now right now, ha ha ha!"
Manic	"I *am* Mistah F. A. B. I'm the hyphiest motherfucking ghost-rider in West Oak. I'm gonna buy this Lexus with my credit card and ghost-ride *that*."
Psychotic	"A tribe of angels is watching me ghost-ride the whip, and Satan is broadcasting the lyrics to *Ghost-Ride It* directly into my brain."
Unhyphy	"Dude, I just wanna park somewhere and get a Slurpee."
Depressed	"Watching YouTube videos of people ghostin' makes me incredibly sad."
Hella Depressed	"I haven't gotten out of bed in a week because all I can think about is how horrible my life is compared to Mistah F. A. B.'s."
Suicidal	"I've said goodbye to my family and friends and am actively seeking out people to roll their car over me as they dance on the hood."

As you can see, there's a broad behavioral spectrum to ghost-riding the whip, and in this case, I've categorized behaviors as "manic" or "depressed" based on how far they deviate from the hypothetical Mistah F.A.B.'s normal hyphy or unhyphy mood states. In the following section, I'm going to be discussing the criteria physicians use to identify the different aspects of bipolar disorder as outlined in the *DSM-IV*, that big fat book published by the American Psychiatric Association that contains the diagnostic criteria for all the psychiatric disorders our society currently believes in. Like the songs in a jukebox, the stock of "mental disorders" in the *DSM* changes all the time—up until 1973, homosexuality was listed as a mental disorder (message to APA pre-1973: y'all must have been tripping *hard*). It hardly needs saying that the *DSM-IV* is not a perfect guide to mental illness, and that some of the "illnesses" that have been described there in the past are no longer considered illnesses at all. Unlike pregnancy, you can't pee on a stick to find out if you have bipolar disorder. Definitions evolve over time, and in a hundred years, the category "bipolar disorder" might be as antiquated as the category "hysteria" is today. The purpose of the following section is to discuss the common symptoms of mania, hypomania, and depression and what they can feel like—and also to help you resist the urge to dump every experience in your life into one of those categories.

NORMAL HAPPINESS AND NORMAL ENERGY—HUZZAH!

When you've just been diagnosed with a major disorder like bipolar, you might have the urge to reinterpret *everything* in terms of either mania/hypomania or depression. But honestly, not every moment in your life is depressed or manic: much of the time, you're just plain old you. Normal happiness and energy are just that—*normal.* You don't need to pathologize your enthusiasm for flying kites or attribute your last romantic success to hypomania. You're probably a charming, loveable, energetic person in "real life"—good for you! You can be ambitious, adventurous, and fun loving outside of mania. The key difference between a "normal" state and a manic or hypomanic state is whether or not your perceptions of reality and your own abilities have shifted, and whether this shift messes up your ability to relate to other people or get your work done. If you're normally a beast on the dance floor who loves to hook up with hot strangers, good for you (enjoy herpes)! If you're a lifelong wallflower who is suddenly electrified with the belief that you're Justin Timberlake bringing sexxy back—well, maybe that's not normal. Let's be perfectly clear: you're allowed to grow and change, try new things, whatever. If done with a clear mind, almost any action you undertake can be considered normal. You should worry about it only if you start basing your actions on unusual logic or logic radically different than your default setting, or if people around you start noticing a marked departure from your usual behavior.

Going skydiving because you think it's cool = normal. Going skydiving *because you temporarily believe you're an invincible god* = not normal. Being a talkative person = normal. All your friend are staring at you because you've been talking like an auctioneer all day = not normal.

MANIA

All ghostin' aside, what is mania, and how can you or other people tell if you're manic? You're manic if your belief about your own capacities expands drastically, if you start engaging in activities that are drastically out of character, making plans drastically out of sync with reality, or behaving in an overblown, irrational, out-of-control manner. It can be hard for *you* to tell if you're manic, at least immediately, but it's pretty easy for other people to tell. You think you're a celebrity, believe you can walk in front of traffic, and obsessively call the Federal Reserve to tell them your brilliant solution to the economic recession. You feel like you don't need to eat or sleep, and feel a vast and potent connection to complete strangers. Words tumble out of your mouth in a great flood. You start taking your job as a mall cop too seriously and stay up all night drafting a new and improved plan for mall safety, which you work on tirelessly with no breaks for several days. *It's the key, the key. People spend all their time in malls, right? Safety is key, right? Mall safety, that's where it's at, that's where it's at.* Your friends and family notice a difference and try to talk you down. "Dear, can we not talk about the menace of escalators tonight?"

Technically, mania is defined by the *DSM-IV* as "a distinct period of abnormally and persistently elevated, expansive, or irritable mood, lasting at least one week (or any duration if hospitalization is necessary)." Therefore, drinking too much coffee and running around like a ferret for *one* day doesn't qualify as a manic episode (unless you get caught by animal control and hospitalized for it). The *DSM-IV* lists seven symptoms of mania, at least four of which are usually present in a full-blown manic episode:[1]

1. *Inflated self-esteem or grandiosity*

   You (mistakenly) think you're famous and important or think you have special powers. You suddenly realize you're a better painter than anyone else in your art class, and start plotting an elaborate gallery opening at the Museum of Modern Art, featuring your work next to Van Gogh's. Your teacher is confused because this represents a major change from your normally humble personality.

2. *Decreased need for sleep*

   You keep coming home from the bar at 3 a.m. Tonight you take a one-hour nap, then go for a run, paint the house, and organize a dinner party for all your friends. Sleep is a bad word.

3. *More talkative than usual*

   You have pressured speech (the sensation that you need to be talking) and a flood of ideas you need to express. Friends and teachers ask you to slow down and explain your thoughts, but it's too hard.

4. *Flight of ideas, racing thoughts*

   Your mind is like a speeding train, or several speeding trains on different tracks. You can't slow down your thoughts, and your ideas fly to their wildest conclusions. You might enjoy the sensation of being flooded with ideas at first, but later become overwhelmed and terrified by it.

5. *Distractibility*

   What?

---

1 *DSM-IV* (American Psychiatric Association [*DSM-IV-TR*], 2000).

6. *Increase in goal-setting activity or psychomotor agitation*

   You're working on a very important project and realize there are three other side projects you should be doing to really get it working. You check twenty books out of the library and start researching every aspect of your subject area. You don't understand why other people can't see the importance of your project. You feel the need to move around a lot.

7. *Excessive involvement in pleasurable activities (such as buying sprees, sexual indiscretions, or foolish business investments)*

   You run to the bar and make out with three different people over the course of a Rihanna single. You buy everyone a round, then flag down a taxi and give the driver a $100 tip for driving you home. You want to buy expensive presents for everybody you know.

The *DSM-IV* definition goes on to state that the above symptoms should not be the result of illegal drugs and must be severe enough to really wreck havoc on your normal life. Psychosis is sometimes a feature of manic episodes, too.

Everyone's experience of mania is different. Some people experience it as a fabulous period of elation, while other people get extremely agitated and experience no pleasure at all. Mania is on a continuum—it takes your normal behaviors and personality and amplifies them. A manic episode can lead to hospitalization or self-harm, and the tomfoolery you get up to while manic can demolish your savings, land you in prison, and make you feel embarrassed later on. Mania can also give you a unique drive and a window into realms of the mind that are inaccessible to most people. In other cultures, mania might be given a different name and be seen as a religious experience. The important thing isn't definitions, which change over time, but *effects*, which vary from person to person. For some people, mania has the effect of a revelation or mystical experience, while for others it only causes misery.

PUTTING IT ALL TOGETHER

Here's how mania might look. The numbers below refer to the symptoms listed on pages 34 and 35.

Let's say you work at a call center for IBM. You spend all day on the phone to customers, helping them fix their computer problems. You're also in charge of logging their questions and complaints in a database. Over the course of a week, you start to notice connections between calls that you never noticed before (4). You realize there's a pattern to the database that could revolutionize the future of IBM (1). You start staying at the office long past closing time, working on solving this pattern far into the wee hours (6). Solving the pattern is more important than eating or sleeping (2). When you tell your coworkers and supervisors about the pattern you discovered, they seem confused, though you talk about it incessantly (3). You get frustrated because nobody else can see how important and revolutionary your discovery is. Even your girlfriend doesn't understand your great discovery, but she wants you to tell Dr. Brunner about it because she thinks he will.

HYPOMANIA

For hypomania, take the mania section and turn the volume down several notches. You talk faster, walk faster, and think faster—enough for other people to comment. Maybe you start writing a novel, building a sailboat, and recording an electro album all on the same day. Or you join a rock-climbing gym because you "suddenly" realize you'd make a fabulous rock climber. It's hard to sleep and hard to sit still and listen when someone else is talking. Other people seem to be talking and moving incredibly slowly. Sitting in class is torture because it seems to drag on for hours and hours, and you've got more important things to do! You might be agitated and elated at the same time, the life of the party, but your engine's running a little hot. You dance down the street, filled with this wonderful sense of how happy the world is, or flit around your room like a trapped fly.

The *DSM-IV* definition of hypomania includes the same seven symptoms as for mania, but the difference is that the episode is not severe enough to land you in the hospital or make it impossible for you to get through a normal day at work or school. It also notes that a change in your mood and behavior should be observable to other people (i.e., that your parents or friends notice that you're talking faster and making uncharacteristic judgments). A hypomanic episode marks a distinct change from your usual self, and the elevated, expansive, or irritated mood should last for at least four days. Hypomania usually isn't accompanied by psychosis, and it doesn't count (at least, not to the guy in the white coat) if your symptoms are due to your taking a drug like ecstasy.

There have been a few books published recently that discuss the advantages of hypomania. *The Hypomanic Edge* by John Gardner and *Finding Your Bipolar Muse* by

Lana Castle both discuss how one can safely harness hypomania to increase one's productivity, creative output, and potential to become a railway tycoon, dominatrix, or Zamboni driver. (OK, I made up the last three, but if I wrote a book about hypomania, those would get at least a chapter each.) Hypomania can imbue you with wonderful feelings of confidence, talent, creativity, self-esteem, charm, and intelligence, all of which can help you achieve great things. It can also feel distinctly uncomfortable and irritating—sometimes both at once. When I'm hypomanic, I love to go running because the pleasure of flying over the pavement is enhanced a million percent. But sometimes underneath the pleasure there's the churning of this desperate engine that wants to go ever faster, and I can't always keep up.

HOW MIGHT MY FRIENDS REACT TO MANIA OR HYPOMANIA?

A good way to gauge whether or not you're acting abnormally is to pay attention to your friends' and family's reactions. Sometimes, nobody will realize you're manic until it's too late. But people who know you can usually sense when something is a little off. From a friend's perspective, your "perfectly reasonable" obsession with the pattern in the IBM call database is *not* perfectly reasonable. A friend can have good insight even when you've lost it. Here are some comments friends might make if you're acting unusually, even if they don't know you have bipolar disorder.

"You're acting really intense."

"You've been working on that project nonstop for a week. Don't you ever sleep?"

"Are you high?"

"What are you talking about? You're not the CEO of Microsoft!"

"Slow down, you're not making sense."

"Are you drunk?"

If friends *know* you have bipolar disorder, they might give feedback like:

"You're getting a bit speedy."

"Have you been sleeping?"

"This is really out of character for you."

It can be really annoying to hear these comments, especially if you feel strongly that you're *not* manic or hypomanic. But it's worth being patient with them, because a trusted friend's insight can help you stop an episode before it gets out of hand.

DEPRESSION AND SADNESS: WHAT'S THE DIFF?

A bunch of nerds had a conference in Las Vegas. After enjoying steak and strippers, they defined clinical depression as having a handful of symptoms that persist for at least two weeks and represent a change from your regular functioning. If you've experienced depression, you can probably list the symptoms yourself: a sad, depressed mood for most of the day; a loss of pleasure in activities you normally like; changes in eating and sleeping; crying a lot; fatigue; recurring thoughts of death. At the extreme, people can become catatonically depressed: too depressed to move or speak. The symptoms of depression overlap with conditions such as vitamin deficiencies and chronic fatigue. So it's important for doctors to rule out other factors when making a diagnosis. Unfortunately, many people with bipolar disorder experience more depressive episodes than manic or hypomanic episodes in their lifetime. How do doctors differentiate between depression and normal sadness or grief? Back to the *DSM-IV!*

1. *Depressed mood most of the day, nearly every day, as indicated by either subjective report (e.g., feels sad or empty) or observation made by others (e.g., appears tearful)*

   You feel sad, down, and empty. Maybe you cry a lot. This feeling persists from day to day.

2. *Markedly diminished interest or pleasure in all, or almost all, activities most of the day, nearly every day (as indicated by either subjective account or observation made by others)*

   You don't feel like going out with friends, doing your laundry, calling your girlfriend, or going to the gym. Activities you normally enjoy feel sad or painful to you.

3. *Significant weight loss when not dieting or weight gain (e.g., a change of more than 5 percent of body weight in a month), or a decrease or increase in appetite nearly every day*

   You find it hard to eat, or you eat a whole box of ice cream just to distract yourself from the sadness. Your body feels strange and makes different hunger demands than usual.

4. *Insomnia or hypersomnia nearly every day*

   You have a terrible time getting or staying asleep at night. Or all you want to do is sleep—you start sleeping twelve hours a day, every day.

5. *Psychomotor agitation or retardation nearly every day (observable by others, no merely subjective feelings of restlessness or being slowed down)*

   You look and feel like you're moving through molasses. It takes you thirty seconds to take your bowl of oatmeal out of the microwave. Your friends get impatient because it takes you forever to put on your jacket. Or you feel agitated and move around like an angry old man.

6. *Fatigue or loss of energy nearly every day*

   You dread the time between periods when you have to walk from one lecture hall to the other. You feel really tired—too tired to do the things you normally do.

7. *Feelings of worthlessness or excessive or inappropriate guilt (which may be delusional) nearly every day (not merely self-reproach or guilt about being sick)*

   You feel extremely guilty about being a terrible friend or being a bad person, for no apparent reason. You feel like you have no worth as a person.

8. *Diminished ability to think or concentrate, or indecisiveness, nearly every day (either by subjective account or as observed by others)*

   You can't make decisions or prioritize tasks. Thinking about whether to go to the bank or the library first nearly kills you. You can't concentrate on a dinner menu, let alone your thesis.

9. *Recurrent thoughts of death (not just fear of dying), recurrent suicidal ideation without a specific plan, or a suicide attempt or a specific plan for committing suicide*

   You can't stop thinking about all things death related. Even if you don't want to commit suicide, you can't stop thinking about how you would do it.

The *DSM-IV* goes on to note the same "ruling-out" clauses as for mania and hypomania: that your symptoms aren't better accounted for by drug abuse, a medical condition like hyperthyroidism or chronic fatigue, or bereavement following the death of a loved one. The depressive symptoms must represent a marked change from your regular functioning and persist over at least two weeks.

The key words are "change from your regular functioning" and "persistent." If you feel like the world has become inherently more depressing and your prospects in life fundamentally bleaker—and these feelings last for a long time and deplete your functioning—it might be depression. If you're just having a bad day and temporarily feel down on yourself, it's probably run-of-the-mill sadness. If you're just not hungry one day, it's probably nothing. But if you lose all desire to eat, have sex, or go outside for two weeks, that's depression. Sometimes you might have a couple days of real depressive symptoms, but manage to pull yourself up before they develop into full-blown depression (tips on doing that later!). In some ways, depression is like the common cold: You can feel it coming on and try to stop it from developing if you catch the symptoms early enough. But once it sinks its teeth in, it can stick around for a long time.

Just like mania, depression can make you do stupid things. On one end of the spectrum, there's suicide, which we'll talk about later. Way on the other end of the spectrum are the stupid thoughts you have when you're depressed. During my last depressive episode, I burst into tears at the sight of a normal white fence and insisted to my boyfriend that it was the saddest fence I'd ever seen in my life. (If you want to see the world's saddest fence for yourself, it's located at 2761 West Seventh Avenue in Vancouver, British Columbia.)

Like hypomania, depression can be harnessed for good. Maybe you take advantage of your reduced energy to spend time reading, or maybe your experiences with depression lead you to write great poetry. Or maybe you embark on a mission to catalogue the world's saddest fences. Who knows?

TRIPPING THE LIGHT PSYCHOTIC

When I first told one of my friends I was taking antipsychotics, she smirked and said, "Oh, you're a psychopath?" Psychosis and "psychotic," its accompanying adjective, are some of the most misused mental-health words out there. First of all, antipsychotics are commonly used for reasons other than psychosis (such as sleep and mood stability), so don't be freaked out if you get prescribed an antipsychotic if you've never been psychotic. Secondly, being psychotic is a totally different thing from being a psychopath. "Psychopathy" means the tendency towards violent, antisocial behavior. Psychosis is when you have delusional beliefs and hallucinations; it can range from experiencing a completely different reality from other people and having no insight, to experiencing voices and visual hallucinations and having some insight into the fact that this experience is not being shared by people around you. Psychosis is on a continuum: some experiences are very close to "normal" reality and some are quite far away.

HALLUCINATIONS

Hallucinations can be auditory, visual, tactile, or even olfactory. You might see people who aren't really there or hear voices giving you commands. Hallucinations can be more or less scary, and they can also be caused by lack of sleep. Like the other aspects of psychosis, hallucinations are on the spectrum of normal human experience and can range from interesting to terrifying and dangerous.

DELUSIONS

Delusions are tricky, because there is such a fine line in our society between which beliefs are considered acceptable and which are considered insane. For example, millions of people hold the same "perfectly normal" religious beliefs that would be considered bizarre and outlandish if they were held by a single person. The *DSM-IV* defines a delusion as "a false belief based on incorrect inference about external reality that is firmly sustained despite what almost everybody else believes and despite what constitutes incontrovertible and obvious proof or evidence to the contrary. The belief is not one ordinarily accepted by other members of the person's culture or subculture." A good example of a delusion is the belief that you're being help captive by kidnappers, when really the "kidnappers" are your stoner roommates who wouldn't even notice if you left the house. If you're delusional, it can be hard to believe friends who tell you your delusions are false. You might believe they're lying, thereby interpreting their comments in a way that confirms your version of reality.

THOUGHT DISORDER

Thought disorder is easiest to identify in a person's speech or writing. It's characterized by a person not making sense from one sentence to the next or making associations that don't make sense to anyone else. For example: "The plane left the airport at three o'clock, and therefore the daisies in the bowl were put there by the dragon."

LACK OF INSIGHT

In psychiatry, insight means the ability to recognize when your behavior and thought patterns are coming from your mental illness as opposed to your regular self. For example: "I realize that the voices in my head aren't coming from real people, even though it really feels like they are."

Insight can vary drastically in psychotic episodes. A person experiencing a full-blown episode of psychosis may not realize that the person sitting next to them on the bus can't also see that the bus is being driven by the Hindu deity Ganesh. Another person experiencing psychosis might slip in and out of insight, alternately realizing that their reality isn't shared and believing that it is. A third person might be aware the whole time that nobody else can see what they're seeing.

In some cultures, what we call psychosis is associated with shamanism and celebrated as a connection with the underworld. I'm just sayin'.

———◆———

Like with any other aspect of bipolar disorder, the boundaries of what we call psychosis are not firmly defined;

what matters most is not how your experience is categorized by the *DSM-IV*, but whether it's having a positive or destructive effect on your life. For example, a lucky person with a great amount of insight, self-discipline, and support from friends and family might be able to treat psychosis as a spiritual experience. For a person who has no support system, no insight, and a comorbidity like substance abuse, psychosis might just be a hellish experience.

OTHER ASPECTS OF BIPOLAR DISORDER

RAPID CYCLING

Rapid cycling means having four or more episodes of mania or depression within a twelve-month period. Rapid cyclers may also have more frequent changes of mood within a week, day, hour, or even minute; the ups and downs are accelerated, and therefore harder to treat. But here's the good news: rapid cycling is not a life sentence. Factors such as drug use and lifestyle can fuel the accelerated cycle of episodes, and a change in lifestyle can significantly slow down the cycles.

MIXED STATES

A mixed state is like a delicious sundae made with both caramel sauce *and* cod liver oil, served on a tantalizing waffle cone of rage. A mixed state is the term for when you experience both manic and depressive symptoms at the same time for at least a week. They generally fall into two categories: dysphoric mania and agitated depression—yin and yang. The former is mania accompanied by things like anger and thoughts of suicide, and the latter is depression with symptoms of hypomania. Not as much is known about mixed states as about vanilla mania or depression, and many people's real experiences of mixed episodes don't meet the diagnostic criteria. Like rapid cycling, this is one of those gray areas that will probably see its definition tweaked a lot over the next hundred years.

CYCLOTHYMIA

Cyclothymia, sometimes referred to as "bipolar lite," is when you have normal moods interspersed with periods of dysthymia (depression too mild too qualify as major depression) and periods of hypomanic symptoms.

"Hey, that sounds like everyone I know. Does the whole world have cyclothymia?"

Not quite. The *DSM-IV* specifies that the symptoms must "cause the patient clinically significant distress or impair work, social, or personal functioning." Furthermore, the euphoric highs and depressive lows in cyclothymia are not in response to life events, but come about for no apparent reason—at least one episode every two months. Cyclothymia sometimes develops into bipolar disorder and, like bipolar disorder, is genetic.

LAST THOUGHTS ON THIS STUFF

Remember, the *DSM-IV* is a tool for categorizing mental illness—not the singular and definitive description of your personal experience. You're a person, not a set of symptoms. When reading this book or any book about bipolar disorder, a "take the best, leave the rest" attitude is in order. Categories and definitions are a lot of cultural flotsam and jetsam that will change with time. The important thing is for you to feel happy, healthy, and cool, no matter what your "diagnosis" is or how the world wants to understand it.

So if any of this technical diagnostic stuff sounds like bullshit to you, just move on down the chapters.

THAT'S SO BIPOLAR: CINDY SHMOE'S GUIDE TO HOW EVERYONE IS, LIKE, SO BIPOLAR

1. OK, so my manager at Tatlow's is, like, so bipolar. One day she's totally nice to me, and the next day she's like, "Why did you dump a pitcher of beer on that guy's head?"

2. Shakespeare prof? Completely bipolar. In class, he's all really energetic and bouncy, and then when I went to pick up my brilliant essay I wrote about how Lady Macbeth is really hearing voices from Joseph Stalin, he acted all sad and depressed.

3. My boyfriend is, like, the most bipolar person I know. When we're out at the club dancing, he looks like he's having such a good time. Then suddenly he gets all mad, and he's like, "Did you just steal my credit card and buy six bottles of hundred-year-old champagne?" And I'm, like, "Obviously."

4. The crazy neighbor lady is such a sad case. I really feel bad for her. She's always coming over to our house to complain about the noise from the building projects I like to do at night. I just hope her kids find her a good rest home.

5. My parents? Bipolarest freaks in town. No, they're both, like, actually bipolar. I'm just glad I don't live with them anymore—it's probably contagious.

3

YOU'VE GOT DRUGS
WRAPPING YOUR HEAD AROUND MEDS

If you've been a happy, healthy person your whole life until coming down with bipolar, suddenly having to take psychiatric medication is a tough pill to swallow. Having bipolar often means taking *meds for life*. Meds for *life*. It takes a while to wrap your head around it. Meds for life makes you realize the severity of the diagnosis. You're suddenly reliant, or expected to be reliant, on these little pills to keep you level and stable. You're not as free anymore: you need your pills. Before, you needed water, air, food, love, and shelter. Now, you need water, air, food, love, shelter, and Risperdal. You'll probably feel disbelief or a yearning for your old freedom and try going off meds again and again to see if you can. In this chapter, we'll talk about the emotions, attitudes, and philosophical perspectives you might grapple with in respect to your medications, as well as what to do if you're prescribed a medication that makes you feel crappy or gives you bad side effects.

WHY MEDS?

Sometimes you can fix your problems by doing yoga, hanging out with different people, doing a ton of creative visualization, and drinking only the purest artisanal "happy" springwater—and sometimes you can't. Taking medication is different from other ways of helping yourself, because medication acts directly on your brain chemistry. It's the fastest way of getting your symptoms under control and the first line of defense against future episodes. Doctors prescribe medications for bipolar because meds produce fast, observable results. Manic person running around psych ward? *Bam!* Meds'll take that sucker down a notch. Depressed person sobbing on couch? *Bam!* Now they're crying in the grocery store aisle. (Meds can help a depressed person regain a little functioning.)

Psychiatric medications have been criticized for this reason: because they work so fast and so effectively, some people fear that they're being used as a replacement for fixing the root causes and behaviors that feed into a mental illness. But medications are also very practical for the same reason: you can't deal with the root causes of your illness if you're too busy being crazy. It's another yin-and-yang situation: meds help you get to a point where you can help yourself in other ways, and helping yourself in other ways can help you be less reliant on meds. Think about your meds as one of several tools you use to create the life you want, rather than a bunch of pills your doctor threw at you to fix you. Don't just take your meds—own them. Understand how they work, why you choose to take them, and what they can and cannot do for you.

Ideally, the purpose of medication is to bring you back to a normal, familiar state of mind—back to your baseline mood. The purpose of medication isn't to change your personality or turn you into someone you're not, but to allow you to be your fullest, happiest self without malfunctioning brain cells getting in the way. The perfect combination of meds should get you to a place where you sigh with relief and say, "I finally feel like myself again!"

I WANT YOU FOR THE REST OF MY LIFE

If you have bipolar disorder, you're probably going to be on medication for the rest of your life. This, perhaps more than anything else, takes a long time to accept. When you're nineteen or twenty, there are very few things you know for sure are going to be with you forever, and you probably didn't think a prescription for antipsychotics was going to be one of them. Well, congratulations newlywed. You and your meds and going to have a long, happy life together. (P.S. I didn't get you anything.)

Taking psychiatric meds for the first time can be a catalyst for thinking about the big questions in life, such as, "What is reality?" and "Who am I?" Are you still authentically *you* when you take mind-altering medication? What about when you have a mind-altering disorder? These are real questions for *everyone*, but for most people, the answers don't affect them in such a concrete way. You're lucky/unlucky enough that you *need* to grapple with these questions because they'll affect real decisions you have to make. Let's examine some beliefs about medication and how they play out with regards to these questions.

BELIEF #1: "BIPOLAR IS A MYSTICAL EXPERIENCE THAT MEDICATION INHIBITS."

It took me three years to really, *really* understand that I was going to need medication long-term. For a long time, it was incomprehensible to me that medication was a real and long-term part of my life. Every few months I'd hide my meds and stop taking them "for good," braving insomnia and other symptoms until I "weakened," gave in, and started them up again. I had a mystical view of bipolar disorder as a fairy-tale challenge I had to overcome. Depression was a deep ocean, and if I could only "get to the bottom of it," it would suddenly dissolve into breathable oxygen. Hypomania was an enchanted forest holding deep wisdom, if only I was fierce enough to push through the brambles. My reasoning? The cycles kept coming back because I refused to really *experience* them. Medication was a way of cheating, of avoiding the final battle with the boss. Like levels in a video game, I had to pass the hardest levels of bipolar disorder, and then I would be done with them forever.

These are important questions: Do mania/hypomania and depression reveal inner wisdom? Do they represent an ultimate experience of grief or ecstasy that will forever be unknown to us if we keep ourselves stable? Do I take medication because I'm too weak, lazy, and scared to confront the powerful experiences I know are lurking just beyond the next tablet? Or is all this mystical thinking a dead end?

External observers (medical researchers, psychiatrists, counselors) note a clear pattern: mood cycles beget mood cycles. You can't prevent future depressive episodes by "getting to the bottom" of your current one. The more you cycle, the bigger the cycles get, and the harder it is to get off the train. The last station is usually a hospital—or worse.

True wisdom is invariant. It's there no matter how you feel or what's going on in the real world. A lot of it is in how you respond to the twists and turns of your mood. Just having depression doesn't make you wise, but calmly weathering it does. Having mania doesn't automatically give you shamanistic powers, but developing insight does. With this in mind, you realize that taking medication doesn't prevent you from having wisdom or an ultimate experience, because those things are created by *you*, not by mania or depression. If some outside force like meds can take away your wisdom, it wasn't real wisdom.

Things to Consider: Do you ascribe a mystical or spiritual element to your bipolar disorder? What's the relationship between spirituality and medication? Is there a mystical aspect to all illnesses or just mental illness?

BELIEF #2: "TAKING MEDS HAS CHANGED WHO I AM."
Grieving for a perceived former self is a normal part of dealing with a bipolar diagnosis. Before, you were healthy, normal, vivid, and emotive. Then suddenly, your wires frayed, and you became, irreversibly, bipolar. Now you

take meds every night. You feel like a different person, in part because you're not having the same moods as before and in part because the old you didn't take meds. Maybe you feel guilty for betraying the old you by subduing her with medication, and you want to let her out. Maybe you're afraid your meds are making you act differently, making you flat or boring. Sometimes they are. (Ask a friend.)

People are very bad at remembering how things really were. It's easier to observe this in, say, some old people, who pine for the good old days when everything was perfect. But it's true for you too. The good old days before you had bipolar sucked a lot too.

This yearning for the pre-bipolar self is an elusive, slippery thing. I've often wondered about it: am I just imagining that I was more brilliant, creative, and authentic before taking psychiatric meds, or was it real? It's convenient to blame a lack of inspiration on meds, but is there also truth in it? When I'm depressed, I long for my happy self. When I'm feeling old, I long for my younger self. It's human nature to think the grass was greener on the other side of the psychiatric fence. And sometimes it really is greener. When you sleep eight hours a night, you lose a certain edge. Even when they hurt, mood cycles make life interesting. Rats have been observed giving themselves electric shocks rather than suffering boredom. When medication makes your mood cycles lose their frequency and intensity, you need to find other sources of magic and foment in your life. You need to find other ways to define yourself and fill your time outside of being manic or depressed.

At the end of the day, only you can decide if being on meds and stable is worth the loss of your old self. But don't make a false god of that old self; chances are that hindsight has bumped it up a few notches from how it really was. And you can never stay the same way forever. Meds or not, you'll keep on growing and changing your whole life.

Things to Consider: What defines an "authentic" experience? Are you authentically you when you're on medication? What about when you're manic or depressed? Do certain medications allow you to feel more like yourself than others?

BELIEF #3: "I MUST BE REALLY WEIRD AND FREAKISH IF I NEED MEDS."

You need meds because you're a creepy, screwed-up freak of nature, right? Otherwise, how do all those people in the world get to sleep without Klonopin or get up in the morning without Epival?

This is a tough part of being diagnosed with a mental illness: the feeling that you're maimed or incompetent in a way that other people are not. In the first few months after I was diagnosed bipolar, I felt like all my friends and roommates could tell I was on medication, even if I hadn't told them, just because it felt like such a big deal to me. I felt ashamed, like I'd been taken down a notch in the world. But over the years, more and more people have come out of the woodwork with their mental illnesses, and it's glaringly obvious that bipolar is due to a roll of the genetic dice, not a failure of character. My boyfriend has a habit of telling people what meds I take, and these days (a few years after diagnosis) it doesn't really bother me. I don't feel like "the strangers" are judging me for "being so weak" anymore.

Millions of people take psychiatric medication at some point in their lives, either long term or temporarily to relieve depression or anxiety. Taking meds has become extraordinarily common, and you probably have friends and relatives who have either taken or are currently taking some kind of psychiatric drug. Sure, an antipsychotic might raise eyebrows more than an antidepressant, but that's because our society still doesn't talk about bipolar and schizophrenia as openly as depression. If you need antipsychotics and your roommate doesn't, it's because the two of you have different genes. Nature's kind of awesome that way.

And even if you were the only person in the world who was being pumped full of meds, well, who cares? It's your life, and if it's better on meds, it's better on meds.

Things to consider: Have you ever talked to your friends and relatives about mental illness? Do you know anyone else on medication? Is it possible to tell when someone is taking psychiatric drugs?

HAWAIIAN VACATION: GOING OFF MEDS

Sometimes, you just wanna go off meds. Life's been boring, and you want something interesting to happen. You wonder if you really need meds anymore; what if you've gotten better? Or you decide meds are making you fat/slow/less creative and throw them down the toilet. (Please don't feed them to your cat/mom/roommate.)

Everybody tries to go off psychiatric meds (except the goody-two-shoes patients that doctors call "compliant"). It's so common it's practically a cliché: I imagine a few years from now there will be a sitcom where the bipolar character is constantly going off his meds and carting expensive modern furniture home to the shared apartment. It's funny to me that, as a population, we consistently try to go off meds and consistently fall on our faces, but keep on trying anyway. It's like we have selective amnesia: each time we fall, we forget about it and try to do the dance again in exactly the same way. Yet for many people (myself included), the urge to go off meds is a crucial part of the bipolar dance.

Why do we try to go off meds? How do we rationalize it? What draws us back to the hot stove each time, while our fingers are still burning from the *last* time we touched it?

Let's rewind forty-odd years to the groovy 1960s, and take a look at this question through the lens of a then-popular theory called Transactional Analysis.

Transactional analysis (TA) is a slightly wacky branch of psychology centered around (you guessed it!) transactions between people. One of TA's central tenets is that in any given situation, a person's primary goal is not to do what will make her happy, but what will reinforce her worldview. The actions and transactions she engages in to reinforce her worldview are called games. For example, a roommate playing the martyr game will stay up after the house party, mop the floor, and pick up all the beer bottles himself—not because it will make him happy, but because it will justify his worldview that he's the only responsible one, and everyone else is a sloppy jerk.

We can think about going off meds as a kind of game—the going-off-meds game, or the "I'm not bipolar, I don't need meds" game. When you try to go off meds, is it because you really believe you'll be a happier, healthier person without them? Or is it because you temporarily have an "I'm not bipolar" worldview that needs reinforcing? One of the crazy things about bipolar disorder is the tricks it plays on your mind, making you think you're better when you're not, or temporarily filling you with disdain for the very treatment that's been keeping your sorry ass out of the hospital for the past six months. Just having bipolar disorder can cause your normal worldview to fluctuate, leading you to play all sorts of games to justify your new worldview. (Parents and significant others, are you listening? Your bipolar kid/boyfriend/girlfriend isn't stupid or crazy for irrationally wanting to go off medication. It's just another aspect of the disorder. Be nice to them.)

Another big idea in TA is that transactions between people are made up of strokes. Think chimpanzees picking through each other's hair for lice. Strokes are the verbal equivalent of petting each other. Different games require different strokes. Think back to the martyr roommate cleaning the kitchen long into the night. Now imagine the following conversation taking place in the kitchen the next morning:

Hungover roommate. Whoa, it's so clean in here.
Martyr roommate, *sighs.* Yep.

Hungover roommate. Did someone, like, stay up all night and clean or something?

Martyr roommate. I did. I was up until 4:30. It took me an hour to get all the vomit out of the couch.

Hungover roommate. Dude, you didn't have to do that. We all would have cleaned today.

Martyr roommate. You always say that, but no one ever does.

Hungover roommate. That's because you always do it before we get the chance.

This situation reinforces the martyr roommate's worldview that his hungover roommate is lazy, that he (martyr roommate) has to do everything himself, and that nobody appreciates him. The martyr roommate sets the game in motion by cleaning up before anyone has a chance to help, thereby ensuring that he will maintain his martyr status. The game winds up with the hungover roommate delivering the strokes ("You cleaned it all by yourself?", "I would have helped!") that the martyr roommate wanted all along.

Going off meds comes with its own set of strokes, or hidden benefits. Maybe the only time you get the attention you crave is when you go off meds, or you only know how to relate to your parents from a position of vulnerability, which you subconsciously seek. Maybe you're uncomfortable or deeply afraid of being stable. Often, people with bipolar disorder simply go off meds because their brain tells them to—it's a compulsion that goes along with the disorder. But if you *do* have insight, you should think about the hidden benefits you're looking for by going off meds, the validity of the worldview you're seeking to reinforce, and consider whether it's really a game you want to play.

GOING OFF MEDS: RISK-REDUCTION-0-RAMA

If you're dead set on a vacation from meds (Hello, future Hilary, are you reading this?), take precautions, because all sorts of things can go wrong, and you could end up dead or in the hospital.

And if you've ever been hospitalized for bipolar disorder, you should never take a medication vacation, even with the precautions I list below. I wrote this section primarily for people with bipolar II, who are at least somewhat less likely to experience major disasters over the course of a few days off meds. I'm not condoning going off meds (are you listening, lawyers?), but since we all know some of us are gonna *try,* we might as well be smart about it.

The precautions boil down to this: make sure somebody you know and trust *knows what you are doing (preeeeferably* a doctor, but honestly, they're going to yell at you, and you want to do something stupid, right?). You need a multiweek "trip sitter." Your trip sitter should be someone who knows you well, is knowledgeable about the symptoms of bipolar disorder, and who either lives with you or is going to check in with you regularly. Best friends and significant others make great trip sitters. Before the start of your med vacation, sit down with this person and hammer out some rules and guidelines for your trip: at what point should the trip sitter encourage you to go back on meds? Are you going to make an agreement to go back on meds if the trip sitter says so? At what point should the trip sitter call your doctor or take you to the hospital? Make sure your trip sitter knows which symptoms to watch for, and that the two of you agree on a plan of action if those symptoms come up. This plan of action is, naturally, only in case of emergency—after all, you don't need meds anymore and you're going to be just fine without them! Right?

I'm going to leave you in charge of your safety and forge ahead with some suggestions from my experience as an experienced/foolish going-off-meds veteran.

- If you decide to go off meds for a while, do yourself a favor and give yourself some wide buffers. For example, if insomnia's a problem, make sure you don't have any classes until after noon. If hypomania's a problem, make sure there's someone checking in with you to make sure you have insight. Don't plan on making any trips or undertaking major activities while you're taking your med vacation.

- Do it "scientifically." Keep a journal of your feelings and observations while you're off the meds. How long do you have to be off meds before you start feeling different? Do you feel different? What's changed? What feels better? What feels worse? At what point do your symptoms start coming back? At what point do you (or your doctor) feel it's really crucial for you to be back on medication? What's the boundary, and which symptoms or behaviors mark this boundary?

- If you believe there's a spiritual element to bipolar disorder, consciously explore it during this time. When you're off meds, do you really feel more spiritual, or were you romanticizing? Are you having the meaningful experiences you thought you would have if you went off meds?

When you go off your meds, you might tell yourself that it's going to be permanent, like going on a diet: "I *swear* I'm never going to eat cake again." But I guarantee you, unless you've been misdiagnosed, you's gonna be back on da crack sooner or later. But don't let that discourage you.

> **Boyfriend,** *deletes "But don't let that discourage you."* You *should* be discouraged. It's a bad idea.
> **Hilary.** What? Why?
> **Boyfriend.** You wrote why earlier. The cycles get worse every time they happ ...
> **Hilary,** *crazy eyes.* But ... you've got to try ... you've *got* to try ...
> **Boyfriend,** *grimaces.*

For some people with bipolar disorder, going off meds has an immediate, nasty, undeniable effect. Other people with bipolar disorder can get through entire months or even years off meds without any symptoms, leading them (OK, me) to believe the whole bipolar diagnosis thing was a huge mistake. Successfully going a month without meds feels, frankly, awesome—like a huge victory. But if you really have bipolar (and weren't misdiagnosed), it's very likely that your symptoms will come back eventually, and the stress the on-meds/off-meds yo-yo puts on your brain chemistry can make future episodes more severe and harder to control.

The times I've gone off meds, my mental narrative was always, "This is the most important thing." I told myself that being off meds was my number-one priority—more important than producing quality work, more important than being a good friend and girl-friend, more important than all the little nuts and bolts that fall to the wayside when I go off meds. But I can never keep up that narrative for long. Within a few days or weeks, I always find something that's *really* more important to me than arbitrarily keeping myself in a state of reduced or altered functioning. For example: "I can't let myself be this wrecked next week, we have to get an issue of the newspaper out!" or "Insomnia is giving me deep spiritual insights, but I'd better sleep so I'm not too cracked out for my date Friday night."

You should think about your priorities. Is the value of being off meds greater than the value of having a stable and productive life? Is being off meds more important than doing well at school or work? Are these mutually exclusive, or can you be off meds and still do all the other things you value? To what extent do your abilities and social relations become impaired when you go off meds? What would cause you to value category "being off meds" above category "getting on with life" or category "tending to things outside myself"? What things in life that you value are still possible when you're off meds? Maybe most of them. Maybe none of them. It's worth thinking about, before you make med vacations a habit.

Last thoughts on going off meds: The value of the often futile exercise of going off meds isn't in finally proving you don't have bipolar (you won't), but in taking careful stock of the things that change or stay the same, why they change, and what you do to support yourself in the absence of meds. When I try to go off meds, I find myself doing all sorts of little things to take care of myself, like going to bed on time and eating well, that I really should be doing year-round. Funny thing.

Things to Consider: Do you wear glasses? Do you sometimes go off wearing glasses for a month to see if your eyesight has fixed itself? Why not? Why is it easy to accept that your farsightedness is real and permanent, but hard to accept bipolar disorder? Can taking medication become as normal and acceptable to you as wearing your glasses?

OBJECTIONS

If you object to taking medication, work through your objections carefully. Are they reasonable, or are they knee-jerk reactions to being told what to do? If you're fearful or suspicious of what taking medication will do to you, talk to your doctor and to other people on psychiatric meds who can address your questions and tell you what it's like for them. As Socrates said, the unexamined life is not worth living—and medication for bipolar disorder should neither be rejected or accepted without a fair trial and serious thought.

People object to taking medication for all sorts of reasons. When it comes to mental illness, some people feel that taking medication is a sign of defeat, weakness of character, or an admission that they really do have a problem. Proponents of psychiatric medication often use the analogy of a broken arm to address those fears: If you have a broken arm, it's not a sign of defeat to put a cast on it. You can't snap out of having a broken arm, so why should you be able to fix depression just by willing it? Of course, the analogy is flawed: a broken arm and bipolar disorder are very different things, with different causes. A broken arm gets fixed once and that's the end of it, whereas a mental illness chugs along for the rest of your life. Broken arms are well understood and don't come with stigma, whereas mental illnesses are fuzzily described at best and heavily stigmatized in our society. Finally, since mental illness lives in the mind, the boundaries between character and illness aren't always clear, which makes people fear that taking medication will screw with their personality.

If you really have a mental illness, you'll have it whether or not you take medication for it; it's not like you're clear up until you pop your first mood stabilizer, at which point you suddenly have a mental illness. If you think taking meds "proves" you have a mental illness, you're like the alcoholic who's afraid to go to AA because it will "prove" he's an alcoholic: you have a mental illness/alcoholism either way, and the only difference is whether or not you're getting help. Putting off taking meds when you need them only lengthens the amount of time you can deny having a problem, not the length of time you have a problem. Thinking of medication in terms of defeat and weakness is a false path, because it mistakenly assumes that not being on medication makes you stronger, smarter, and more honorable.

The truth is, you can be a strong person whether or not you're on meds. True strength is having levelheaded insight into all of your decisions, thoughts, feelings, and reactions—not an arbitrary marker like on meds or off. The severest forms of mental illness rob you of all insight. And if you don't have insight, you have nothing. If you need to be on meds to keep it, so what?

MEDS THAT SUCK

Early on in my bipolar days, the doctor I was seeing prescribed Depakote to get me down from a mild hypomania (induced by the antidepressants she'd prescribed the previous week). Suddenly, my world was flat and dark, unbearable. The brief light I'd glimpsed during the hypomania was choked at the source, and thoughts came slowly and dully. I felt lobotomized. More than that, I felt betrayed—like a bird set free from its cage, only to be shot out of the sky. What had I done to deserve this horrible punishment? I did some online research and when I saw the doctor again, told her I wanted to try a different combination of drugs. She agreed, and within a few weeks I'd found a combination (an antipsychotic and a mood stabilizer) that has more or less worked for me ever since.

At some point during your bipolar career, especially in the beginning when you're trying to figure out which drugs work for you, you might be given a Med That Sucks. This med doesn't suck for everybody (otherwise it wouldn't be on the market), but it sure sucks for you. Taking a Med That Sucks is traumatic. You feel tortured, frantic, and angry at whoever prescribed it. You sure as hell don't plan to take it for the rest of your life.

Go back to your doctor, cry, complain, but don't take this as an opportunity to renounce psychiatric medication for the rest of your life. All meds were not created equal, and it can take a lot of trial and error before you finally hit on a combination of meds that works for you. Remember that time when you were a kid when you got cabbage rolls for dinner and hated them? Did you renounce eating dinner forever? Psychiatric meds are like food when everyone's a picky eater. Be patient. Keep on trying. You'll find something that makes you feel like yourself again.

SIDE EFFECTS

At some point in your bipolar career (maybe now), you might be prescribed a drug that comes along with the miserable gang of gremlins known as side effects. Side effects range in type and severity, from the mildly amusing (excessive drooling) to the deadly (liver failure). Side effects vary from drug class to drug class, but the most common ones across the board are insomnia, drowsiness, weight gain, and sexual dysfunction. Less commonly, psychiatric meds can cause people to develop conditions like tardive dyskinesia (an involuntary twitch) and high cholesterol. And rarely, some sucker will develop the most unlucky side effect of all: death.

When an unbearable side effect crops up, there are a few different courses of action available. Your doctor will either reduce or discontinue your dosage of that drug, replace it with a different drug in the same class, keep you on the offending drug but add another drug to counteract the side effects of the first one, or just encourage you to put up with the side effect without making any changes in your med regime. Which route you take depends on the severity of the side effects as weighed against the risk and hassle of switching meds. For example, if you've already tried every atypical antipsychotic on the planet and the only one that works for you makes you gain ten pounds, the disruption involved in trying out a new slew of drugs might be more trouble than it's worth. If you have uncontrollable leg twitching, on the other hand, you gotta change meds.

Deciding what to do about serious side effects is easy: your doctor will obviously want to treat them or stop prescribing whatever's causing them. Dealing with the lesser, run-of-the-mill side effects is much trickier. Basically, you have determine whether the benefit of the drug outweighs the cost of the side effects, and if a different drug could provide the same benefit minus the side effects. Can you deal with being ten pounds heavier or having a dry mouth sometimes, if it means you're not depressed anymore? Can you handle twitching and drooling your way through law school if it means you don't have another manic episode? It sucks, but sometimes you just need to compromise and hold out for the side effect–free wonder drugs of the future.

IT'S ALL YOU

If you're a miserable jerk, going on psychiatric meds will alleviate your bipolar symptoms, but it won't make you *stop* being a miserable jerk. If you were a happy person before coming down with bipolar, you should still be a happy person on meds. If you were a bitchy, cranky person before being diagnosed bipolar, you'll still be a huge bitch on meds. Medication takes care of the parts of yourself you can't control, like your brain chemistry. Medication will not take care of the things you *can* control, like your worldview, your habits, and your reactions to life events.

Happy people are happy because out of the huge gamut of possible reactions to any given event or situation, they consistently choose the positive ones. If a happy person is starving, her face will shine with anticipation of the next delicious meal. A miserable person, however, will have an inner dialogue focusing on how starving and miserable she is. If a happy person gets diagnosed bipolar, she might be worried about it for a while, but ultimately carry on with a normal, exuberant life. If a miserable person gets bipolar, no amount of medication will make her feel less miserable—less manic, yes, but not less miserable.

Solution? Be aware at all times of the many responses you could have to any situation. As much as you can, choose patience over impatience, calm over frustration, grace over fear, and happiness over disappointment. The decisions you make from moment to moment are more powerful than any medication in determining your overall happiness in life.

4

SHRINKS
WHAT THEY'RE FOR AND HOW THEY CAN HELP

WHY SHRINKS?

In medieval Wales there were poor men and women known as sin-eaters, whose job it was to eat the sins of folks who'd died so the dead person's soul could go to heaven. Their job sucked. The family of the deceased person would pass the sin-eater bread and wine over the coffin to symbolize the transfer of sins from the dead person to the sin-eater. Then the dead person would waltz into heaven, his family would be relieved, and the sin-eater would get a piece of bread and a pile of damnation.

Shrinks are sin-eaters, minus the poverty, coffins, and eternal damnation. They specialize in receiving all your psychic ills—all the dredged-up memories, patterns, abuses, delusions, and baggage you carry around. It's a shrink's job to listen to your stories and ask for more. Because you're paying them top dollar to listen, there's no guilt in talking about yourself for an hour. Unlike unburdening to a best friend, you don't have to worry about your shrink's needs or make sure she's getting enough support from the relationship. She's your sin-eater; your pain is her gain. Because your psychiatrist isn't part of your family or social group, you don't have to worry that anything you say will screw up your relationships or damage anyone's trust in you. She has nothing to lose or gain from anything you say or do, and is, therefore, objective. The client-shrink relationship is, by definition, unbalanced. It's balanced by cash—piles of cold, hard cash. You show up and give your shrink an honest account of your mind, and she listens, guides you to understanding, and prescribes pills to help you out in the afterlife.

Psychiatrists exist to step in when the general population is no longer qualified to deal with your shit. You go to a shrink when:

- *You're manifesting symptoms and behaviors that most nonshrinks can't identify or make sense of.*

  Psychiatrists have seen people like you in patterns like yours hundreds of times. They understand what the "bipolar" pattern looks like and can even predict how it will unfold in the future. Whereas your best friend might love you, but not understand the difference between mania and a caffeine buzz, your shrink doesn't love you (ouch, I said it!), but knows her diagnostic ass from her elbow. She also has studied and, perhaps more important, *seen* the difference between bipolar, taking coke, schizophrenia, alcoholism, and hypochondriacs who love to be diagnosed.

- *You need an objective outsider to talk to.*

  Your struggle with a mental illness can put a lot of stress on your relationships with your family and friends. Even a close friend can only handle so much without feeling drained. On the other hand, you can work through all your toxic baggage with a shrink with no fear of straining or damaging your intimate relationships. Talking to a shrink is cathartic precisely because the shrink is not involved in your life in other ways. Your friends don't even have to know you're seeing one.

- *You need someone to prescribe and monitor your meds.*

Psychiatrists are allowed to prescribe meds and tweak them according to your needs. Of course, you don't to see a psychiatrist every week for as long as you're on psychiatric meds, but if you're still trying to find a combination of drugs that works for you, or if your existing meds suddenly stop working, a psychiatrist will help you get your feet back on solid ground.

The following table highlights the differences between three popular therapeutic options:

	Best Friend	Psychiatrist	Hell's Angels
Experienced with insanity?	Read *Touched With Fire*.	Went to med school, seen a lot of different people.	Yes.
Prescribes drugs?	Can't.	Can.	Lots.
Talk about your problems?	Yes.	Yes.	Favors chain beatings.
Is objective?	Dates your brother.	Doesn't.	Whacked your brother.

FUNCTIONS OF A SHRINK

Now that we've talked about why you might see a shrink, let's take a closer look at the specific functions of a shrink. Outside of abstract notions like healing and catharsis, what are the practical, concrete functions of a psychiatrist or therapist? Which of those functions are unique to licensed therapists/psychiatrists, and which can be filled by free resources like friends, support groups, and books?

Going to a shrink lets you:

- check in with someone.
- talk about yourself and about private, sensitive issues.
- get advice and prescriptions (from psychiatrists only, not psychologists) for your medications.
- see someone who knows when you need hospitalization.
- do something productive that gives you a sense of positive action over your disorder.

Seeing a shrink can also:

- help you gain traction in your life.
- help you understand your diagnosis.
- help you identify maladaptive (counterproductive, negative) thoughts and behaviors and replace them with useful ones.
- act as sounding board for whether certain thoughts or behaviors are irrational.
- help you plan for the future, set goals, and decide on actions to take.
- give you the opportunity to talk about relationships and family stuff with someone who's uninvolved.
- give you a regular, scheduled activity.

Obviously, seeing a psychiatrist isn't the only way to get a regular, scheduled activity into your life or feel like you're being proactive about bipolar. You could just as easily join a bowling league or attend a support group. Have a look at the following table.

Functions of a Psychiatrist	Shrink	Books	Support Group	Free Clinic	Grandma
Listen to your problems	X		X	X	X
Help you understand your diagnosis	X	X	X	X	
Act as a sounding board	X		X	X	X
Help you plan and set goals	X	X		Maybe	X
Help you identify maladaptive behaviors	X	X	Maybe	Maybe	Maybe
Provide you with a regularly scheduled activity	X		X	X	X
Tweak your medication	X				
Give medical advice	X				
Check in with you	X		X	X	X
Be an objective, uninvolved listener	X				

Think about what you want to get out of therapy. Maybe you need short-term help dealing with the emotions that a bipolar diagnosis stirred up. Maybe you're rapid cycling and need to see a psychiatrist long term as you flip through episode after episode and try out different meds. Maybe you're just thinking therapy's sexy and like the idea of having a primal-scream therapist on your roster. Whatever your reason for seeing a shrink, remember that therapy isn't a magic spell or an escape from the world; it's one of many tools you can choose to use (or not) to help you establish a better life with bipolar.

WHAT'S THE DIFFERENCE BETWEEN A PSYCHIATRIST AND A PSYCHOLOGIST?

Psychiatrists are physicians with medical degrees (they have "M.D." after their name). Psychologists (who come in many flavors, which we'll discuss later) have doctorates and training in psychotherapy, but do not have medical degrees. Psychiatrists are doctors of medicine, and clinical psychologists are doctors (in the academic sense) of psychology.

In most states, only psychiatrists are allowed to prescribe medication. This might be changing: in Louisiana and New Mexico, psychologists are now allowed to prescribe meds for mental illnesses, and Oregon recently passed a bill allowing psychologists to prescribe psychotropic drugs only. Whether or not psychologists should be allowed to prescribe drugs is an ongoing debate in the health-care community, with proponents pointing to the fact that it's more efficient for patients to see one shrink who is empowered to prescribe drugs rather than bouncing around between two different shrinks, one of whom can prescribe drugs and one of whom can't. Opponents claim that without med school training in biochemistry, pharmacology, and physiology, psychologists can't safely prescribe powerful psychotropic drugs.

Anyway, point is, many people with bipolar disorder see both a psychiatrist *and* a clinical psychologist or another kind of therapist. Talk about double-fisting!

SEND IN THE CLOWNS: THERAPY OPTIONS

Now let's have a look at a handful of different therapy options and their pros and cons. Send in the clowns!

CLOWN #1: PSYCHIATRIST

A typical session with a psychiatrist is about an hour long. Like your family doctor, she'll start off the first session by asking about your family history, medical/psychiatric history, current life circumstances, and the events that precipitated your coming in to see her. Then she'll move into psychiatrist territory, asking questions about your moods, energy levels, how much sleep you're getting, what your day-to-day life is like, and your relationships with your family, friends, and/or partner. She'll also want to know about your past: Did you have a happy childhood? Did you enjoy high school? How old were you when you started drinking, having sex, doing drugs, etc.? The psychiatrist wants to figure out certain things about you: how you deal with stress, how you view yourself in the world, how you relate to other people, and how you relate to important events in your past. If there are any specific issues going on in your life, this is the time and place to talk about them in as much depth as you need.

A good psychiatrist will also help you understand your diagnosis and help you develop strategies for avoiding future episodes. If you keep seeing a psychiatrist over an extended period of time, she'll probably get the chance to observe you in a number of different states: from really depressed to baseline to kinda speedy. Your psychiatrist is also in charge of prescribing medication and monitoring its effects on you (to the extent that she has the opportunity to observe you) and is the person to talk to about making any tweaks to your med regimen.

Good for you if: you need someone to prescribe psychiatric meds, you have life events (such as childhood abuse) you want to talk about, you want someone to check in with on a regular basis, you have a lot of questions about bipolar disorder and medication.

Not the ideal fit if: you hate the idea of talking about yourself for an hour, you feel like you have "nothing to talk about," you see traditional psychiatry as "the Man."

CLOWN #2: COGNITIVE BEHAVIORAL THERAPIST

A cognitive behavioral therapist has an advanced degree in either psychology or social work, and may also be certified by the National Association of Cognitive Behavioral Therapists (NACBT). Cognitive-behavioral therapy (CBT) is the most concrete, action-based of the psychotherapies. The therapist helps you identify which thoughts and behaviors are bringing you down, and gives you specific tasks to do to fix them. The purpose of CBT is to help you become your own therapist. Therefore, you usually plan to see a cognitive-behavioral therapist twelve to eighteen times, not indefinitely, because after a number of sessions you've hopefully developed enough skill to help yourself without regular visits to the therapist. The heart and soul of CBT is helping you identify thought patterns, behaviors, and assumptions you hold that may be reinforcing your difficulties. For example, if you deal with stress by getting angry at other people, the therapist will help you develop a new, healthier thought pattern. CBT tends to be heavy on homework. Between sessions, you'll probably have to keep a journal of stressful situations and your reactions to them, and your therapist will also give you a weekly task or experiment to complete. Pure CBT is not so much about mulling over your past and gaining insight into your subconscious as it is about taking practical, immediate action to challenge your maladaptive (read: counterproductive) behaviors. During a CBT session, you'll review your homework, set new homework, and maybe do some role playing or visualization to practice your new responses to stressful situations.

Good for you if: you want to address a specific problem (e.g., shyness, self-injury, low self-esteem, troubled relationships), you're looking for self-empowerment, and you respond well to goal-setting activities.

Not the ideal fit if: you don't have a specific issue to work on, you just need someone to talk to, you don't want to do homework between therapy sessions.

CLOWN #3: INTERPERSONAL AND SOCIAL RHYTHM THERAPIST

This clown is another kind of psychologist, with an advanced degree in psychology or social work. Interpersonal and Social Rhythm Therapy, or ISRT, targets your circadian and social rhythms in order to stabilize your bipolar disorder. An ISR therapist takes a look at everything you do in a typical day and when you do it: what time you wake up, what times you eat, what times you engage in social interaction, what time you work, what time you exercise, etc. The purpose is to help you establish the best possible rhythm of life. Interestingly, ISRT is one of the only therapies shown to be effective in treating bipolar disorder specifically. Since a big part of bipolar disorder is having your rhythm of life disrupted—for example, by insomnia, hyperactivity, and elevated or reduced desire for social interaction—ISRT researchers have found that tweaking and stabilizing your patterns of social interaction can have a real stabilizing effect on your mood. During a typical ISRT session, you'll look over the records of activity you made that week and your resulting moods. For example, you might determine that you should be getting up earlier and exercising in the morning rather than at night, or that you feel happiest when you make your first social contact of the day no later than 1 p.m. As IRST is a relatively recent (and promising!) development in psychiatry, it might be hard to find a counseling center in your area.

Good for you if: you're a nerdy, practical type who's up on your game and interested in cutting-edge bipolar research, you could benefit from a therapeutically approved schedule, you want a way to prevent future episodes.

Not the ideal fit if: you're never going to follow the improved rhythm you and your therapist come up with, you hate schedules and are married to having an erratic lifestyle, you want insight and healing to traumatic events, not lifestyle solutions.

CLOWN #4: PSYCHOANALYST

A psychoanalyst may or may not have an advanced degree in psychology or social work (or indeed, any kind of degree. More on that later). The most glamorous of the therapies, psychoanalysis is also the most spooky. The psychoanalyst's job is to help you uncover your unconscious motivations. That's where the stereotype of "I can't figure out how to work the mail machine because Daddy never loved me" comes from. During a typical psychoanalysis session, you might talk about your dreams, play a free-association game, and discuss your relationship to the psychoanalyst herself. One of the main ideas of psychoanalysis is that your relationship to your analyst mirrors your relationship to other important people in your life. So if you feel fearful and angry towards your analyst, it might indicate fear and anger towards, say, your father. Psychoanalysis also emphasizes understanding how events in your past are getting played out in the present, and helping you move beyond traumatic experiences.

Warning: The term "psychoanalyst" is not regulated by the federal government or by most states. That means anyone can legally call herself a psychoanalyst (even me. That will be $150 an hour, please!) Look for a psychoanalyst who has been certified by the American Psychoanalytic Association—they receive rigorous clinical training and have either medical degrees or advanced degrees in psychology or social work.

Good for you if: you're interested in the subconscious, you have important relationships you need to work out, you're into Freud, you've done your research.

Not the ideal fit if: you think Freud's theories are bogus, you hate analyzing things, you want a traditional kind of therapy approved by modern medicine.

MALL CLOWN: LIFE COACH

Life coaches are not medical professionals and don't necessarily have degrees in psychology, but I include them here because some family doctors recommend life coaching to their patients and because they're a cheaper option than psychiatrists if all you need is help getting organized and determining your goals.

Life coaches come in many flavors. Some specialize in career coaching, some in life skills like how to go grocery shopping, and some will even help you become a dream date. A life coach's job is to help you clarify your needs and to set and achieve clear goals in any number of areas (relationship, job, school, personal). If you're confused about where you're going in life or what you should be doing, a good life coach will know just the right questions to ask to get you to that a-ha! moment when you realize your purpose in life (or your purpose this week). Like cognitive-behavioral therapy, life coaching is very action oriented: you will leave the session each week with a set of tasks to carry out that will get you closer to your goals. Sometimes, life coaches are recommended to people who just don't know how to get started on a particular task, like applying for college.

Life coaches are not professionally licensed, like therapists or psychiatrists. In fact, life coaching is a completely unregulated field. That means *anyone* can legally call themselves a life coach with absolutely no training, certification, or supervision. They can't prescribe medication, give psychiatric advice, or deal with things like psychosis. While awesome, sincere, committed life coaches do exist, there are plenty of unqualified "life coaches" out there who will take your money and send you home with a photocopied list of canned "affirmations" to stick on your fridge, leaving you no better equipped to deal with your life.

Good for you if: you need someone to help you get your life on track in a basic way, you need help identifying your goals and making a strategy to achieve them, you want someone who's "on your team" to act as a sounding board, you're basically stable and don't need the psychiatric services of a therapist.

Not the best fit if: you need someone who can give psychiatric counseling and medical advice (a life coach is *not* a therapist), you want to discuss your past and relationships, you need something more than help with life goals.

KID'S BIRTHDAY PARTY CLOWNS: ALTERNATIVE THERAPISTS

In addition to the five well-known flavors of mind-helpers described above, you might also hear of alternatives like somatic therapy, art therapy, music therapy, and play therapy. These therapists use activities like drumming, painting, guided visualizations, body awareness, and acting out your dreams with toys to help you gain insight and heal your psychic wounds. Alternative therapists are sometimes less expensive to see than psychiatrists, or they might charge on a sliding scale.

The measure of these alternative therapies, like the measure of the mainstream ones, is whether or not they work. Ask yourself: Does this therapy leave me better equipped to deal with my life? Does this therapy help me gain insight into my thoughts, behaviors, and disorder? Is this therapy helping me move forward? If the answer is "yes," then it doesn't matter whether the therapy is mainstream or "alternative"— it's working for you!

When any kind of therapy ceases to do the above things, you're finished. When you go into a therapy session and have absolutely nothing left to say, you're finished. When you feel like a totally stable, cool person on good terms with being bipolar, you're finished. If something comes up down the road, you can always go back.

CLOWN Q&A

In the rest of this chapter, I'll answer gnarly shrink-related questions like, "Can I lie to my shrink?" "What's it like attending a support group?" and "What's it like being hospitalized for bipolar?"

"CAN THE CLOWN TELL IF I'M LYING?"

Depends on the clown, how good a liar you are, and whether or not you secretly want the shrink to know you're lying (as people who lie often do). Of course, it's more useful to you if you *don't* lie to your shrink. What's the point of paying someone to help you if you won't give them the right tools by telling the truth? Remember, you're hiring *them* to help *you*. You don't have to be ashamed of anything, and an honest relationship with someone whose professional duty it is to be nonjudgmental isn't something to throw away lightly. Besides, she can usually tell.

Once I decided to hitchhike to San Francisco over Christmas break with a boy I was intrigued by, but felt my plan was too complicated to explain to my psychiatrist when she inquired about my holiday plans. The scenario went like this:

> **Shrink.** What are your plans for Christmas break? Are you going to see your family?
>
> **Hilary.** No, I'm going to San Francisco with a guy I met in the Varsity Outdoors Club.
>
> **Shrink.** How are you getting there?
>
> **Hilary,** *shifty eyes.* Dri-i-i-ving.
>
> **Shrink.** Does your boyfriend know this guy?
>
> **Hilary,** *shifty eyes.* Y-e-e-e-s.
>
> **Shrink.** Ah.

You lie to your shrink because you don't want her to make a big deal about something, you don't want to retard your progress by admitting something touchy, or you want to be done with therapy and therefore don't want to bring up any new issues. These are all valid reasons. But when your shrink asks if anything's come up in your life, it's easier just to say, "My dog died, but I'm cool with it," than to say nothing's happened and make her think you're hiding something.

In my book, support groups fall under the category of shrink-like because you're talking to a bunch of strangers who have a lot of experience with bipolar and who can help you figure out if what you're experiencing is crazy or not. They're the next best thing to talking to a therapist. But going to a support group for the first time feels even weirder than going to a psychiatrist, because you wonder if you've joined the icky underclass of watery-eyed, rambling narcissists you see on TV. It's one thing to visit the circus, it's another thing to attend a clown convention. You feel like just showing up to a support group taints you as defective, "one of them." You don't want to identify with those people. It's too bad we have those fears, because bipolar support groups—particularly, support groups for young people with bipolar—can be awesome.

Many cities in the United States and Canada have support groups sponsored by the Depression Bipolar Support Alliance (DBSA), or by the National Alliance on Mental Illness (NAMI). Here's what it's like to attend a typical DBSA-sponsored bipolar support group.

You go to a meeting room and sit in a circle on plastic chairs. There might be anywhere from two to twenty other people there, plus a moderator. They're normal people—the kind of people who sit next to you in class or come into the coffee shop where you work. The moderator reads the rules: everything's confidential, no swearing or violence, "We're not doctors, we can't give you medical advice, don't sue us." Then you go around the circle, and when it's your turn, you say your name, which meds you're on, and what issue you want to talk about. Examples of typical issues people bring to support-group meetings are:

"I hate my meds."

"I'm really depressed."

"Does this particular thought/behavior/experience sound manic to you?"

"Does this particular thought/behavior/experience sound paranoid or psychotic to you?"

"I'm having a problem with my friends/parents."

"How do I cope with …?"

The first time I went to a support group, I got really stressed out trying to think of an issue. I was doing fine, and I didn't feel like I had anything serious enough to merit discussion. But since everyone else in the group had something big to talk about, I fished out a story about being hypomanic and responding to a Craigslist ad looking for actresses for a "feminist erotic movie." I didn't end up acting in any movies (much to everyone's relief who had heard my bright-eyed plotting when I was hypomanic), but I'd called the phone number and met up with a curly-haired European porn director in an Oakland pizza restaurant, feeling very glamorous and risqué. It had taken a lot of high-octane convincing from my boyfriend to make me sleep on it for a few nights before going any further. My "issue," I explained fumblingly, was figuring out whether I really wanted to be a feminist soft-porn actress or if it was just hypomania. When I finished my story, the moderator made a few general comments about hypomania, then asked if I had problems with chronic lying.

This is one of the downsides of support groups: you can feel pressured to present something crazy enough to deserve support, and other participants can feel pressured to interpret everything you say in a bipolar light. The support-group setting can lead everyone to overpresent and overrespond. A good support-group moderator will counteract this effect by encouraging honest interactions and a certain amount of casual conversation amid the bipolar talk. But a bad moderator will compound this effect by divining a pathological, bipolar reason for everything you say and do. With this warning in mind, you should be able to tell a good or bad support group when you see one.

Ideally, a support group is an arena in which you have full license to talk about your bipolar-related issues with people who have similar experiences and a sounding board against which to check if you're acting strangely. Plus, the people in the support group aren't part of your family or social crew, so they have the bonus of uninvolvement (or as much involvement as you choose to grant them).

Last thoughts on support groups:

- Just because you attended a certain group once doesn't mean you're committed to going every time. Shop around until you find one that makes you feel less crazy, not more crazy.

- Support groups exist for *you*. If the format is ineffective, suggest ways to make it better. People have a tendency to passively stick with a particular system just because it's there. Be a mover and shaker—make it better!

- Consider trying out a support group even if you're completely stable and happy. It can be fun to meet other people with bipolar disorder, and that way you'll already have a larger support system to draw on when you *do* have problems.

"WHAT'S IT LIKE BEING HOSPITALIZED?"

You don't have to go further than the local library or video store to find accounts of life in the psych ward. Accounts of hospitalization for mental illness are often poeticized, dramatized, and scandalized—and with good reason. Crazy shit goes down in psych wards— that's what psych wards are *for*—but not crazy in the fun way. People who have been there will tell you very firmly that you do *not* want to be hospitalized. It's not glamorous, sexy, or fun in any way. It won't give you mystique or higher cred with your bipolar homeboys or homegirls. Doctors hate hospitalizing people, especially young people, because a one-week hospitalization can set you back an entire year. It ain't worth it.

The how's and why's of hospitalization for bipolar vary from case to case. If you really went wild and got fifty-one fiftied, your memory of the first few days of hospitalization will be hazy with sedation. If you're only "pretty manic" and check yourself into an institution, you'll come out with clearer memories of what exactly went down while you were there. Either way, life on the psych ward isn't a barrel of laughs. You see doctors. You hang out in the dayroom watching TV. You get a bit of exercise walking up and down the hall or playing Ping-Pong. You spend a lot of time waiting for your next meal. There might be group-therapy sessions or outings to the ice cream parlor, and visits from your parents or friends. A hospitalization can last anywhere from a few

Joshua Walters, now twenty-four, was hospitalized three times between ages sixteen and eighteen. He describes the experience of hospitalization as a time of confusion, boredom, and longing to get out. The adult ward on which he was placed during his second hospitalization consisted of a windowless unit with a long hallway where the patients would walk up and down for exercise: "You had the TV and the room to eat in and then you had this hallway where people would just walk up and down, and that was your day."

Heavily sedated, he spent the hours between mealtimes writing, playing board games, or watching TV.

"Your whole day is centered around meals, because you're not doing anything. You're not working. You're not even relaxing. You're just there. They don't know what to do with you, you're just there until you get better," he said.

After a few days of confusion following his psychotic break, Joshua figured out where he was and grew determined to get out—a challenging process.

"The thing is," he explains, "in a room full of loonies and people who are really crazy, you have no example for sanity. You have the nurses who are, like, 'Take your medicine,'" and chasing after you, but there's no example for, 'Hey, you know, you should try [acting] like this to get out of the hospital.'" He later figured out that one of the men on the ward, who dressed in normal clothing and acted calmly, was actually a hospital staff member whose job was to provide an example of "normal" behavior.

After two weeks on the ward, Joshua improved enough to be let out. He says of hospitalization, "After that happens, you make it a promise to yourself that you will never go back there, because of how alienating the experience is to you and how you're removed from your life."

nights to years, but for a manic episode, it's usually a few weeks.

That's it.

"WHAT IF I WANT THERAPY BUT CAN'T AFFORD IT?"

If your health insurance doesn't cover therapy, don't despair, for the following reasons:

- Therapy alone isn't effective at treating bipolar disorder. Tons of people (myself included) get along just fine without it. But if you really need it, and you can't get it, proceed to the next option.

- Many cities have free counseling centers or clinics that offer sliding-scale payment options. For example, at the Integral Institute in San Francisco, you can get a session with a therapist for as little as ten dollars. Some free clinics have "real" therapists, and some have trained volunteer counselors. Obviously, volunteer counselors are unable to give medical advice or prescribe medication, but they can fulfill the therapist's function of checking in with you, giving feedback, and providing you with a safe space to talk about your issues. Free clinics and alternative counseling centers can be a bit of a grab bag in terms of quality, but if you think about the *function* of therapy, rather than the form it takes, you can see how a combination of free resources can add up to the value of for-payment therapy. By the way, support groups fall into the category of free resources that are "like therapy." If you're a college student, your college or university might also have a free psychiatrist on call during certain hours.

CONCLUSION

The world of psychiatrists, therapists, support groups, and hospitals can be really daunting when you first fall into it. Trying out all these shrinks and shrink-like activities can make you feel crazier than you really are, especially if you go into it with a lot of fears and anxieties about what seeing a shrink or attending a support group says about you. As you get more familiar with the bipolar game, it will stop feeling so weird, and you'll start to see yourself on a more equal playing field with your options. You start to realize you don't see a psychiatrist "because you're crazy"; you see a psychiatrist because you happen to get x and y benefits out of seeing a psychiatrist. You don't go to a support group because you're a loser; you go because it's fun and useful to talk to other people who've been where you are. Think of everything in terms of its effect—what it *does* for you, not what it "makes" you.

5

THIS IS YOUR MANAGER SPEAKING
TAMING EPISODES WITH FOOD, SLEEP, AND EXERCISE

It's good to be a robot! Programming yourself into positive exercise, eating, and sleeping habits can have a more profound effect on your mood than any drug. This chapter is all about taking the bipolar bull by the horns and taming it with a little oatmeal and Tae Bo.

Anyone who's had a repetitive food-service job knows the drill. You prep the food, wipe the counters, make change for people, and eat the odd avocado that "fell on the floor." Eventually, working in Bob's Taco Shack becomes second nature to you. Like it or not, it's your job, and if you don't do it well, Bob's gonna kick your ass back to your parents' basement in Kansas. Taking good care of your bipolar self is the same thing: a job. But instead of monitoring the tomato-to-onion ratio in the salsa, you've got to monitor your stress levels and develop good habits and routines. The three top tools with which you can effectively do this are exercise, nutrition, and sleep. Congratulations, Sparky, you've just been promoted to manager.

WHAT IS A MANAGER?

Your manager is you at your most loving and responsible, the you who looks out for the you at your most depressed or manic. It's the voice in your head that remains objective, insightful, and on the ball even when the "real you" feels despairing or out of touch. When depressed you feels like bingeing on beer and hookers to cure your depression, your manager suggests a bowl of oatmeal. When manic you is freaking out because the king of Thailand didn't write back to your e-mail, your manager keeps you company and takes you for walks until you feel better. Your manager's not a nasty or dictatorial voice, but a friend that swoops in to help you in times of need. Read on to see what kinds of habits your manager can help you establish.

EXERCISE

When I was diagnosed with bipolar, I joined a women's gym for the express purpose of crying in the showers. I kept the gym a secret and went there whenever I needed to escape from my regular haunts. Six months later I had not only set the record for longest showers taken by any gym member, but I also had inadvertently developed lungs of iron and abs of steel. Or abs of tinfoil. Whatever. Point is, exercise is good for all sorts of things beyond just getting in shape. It gets you out of the house. It burns off excess energy. It distracts you from your problems. It can give you some fine people-watching and/or people-meeting experiences. It floods your body with happiness-inducing endorphins. And it can require as little or as much mental sharpness as you have to spare. As my friend says about her solo swimming habit, "No matter how crazy I feel, it all levels out in the pool. The water stays the same whether I'm depressed or not, and somehow that makes me feel better."

All exercise is not created equal, and while benefits overlap across the spectrum, different activities suit different moods. An activity that can be done solo, like running or swimming, can see you through misanthropic periods, while team sports like basketball and soccer can help you build a social network and give you a reason to leave your house on Wednesday nights. Then there's rhythmic, sustained exercise, like cycling, versus sports involving sudden bursts of energy, like tennis.

People with depression and bipolar benefit from exercise that involves a sustained, repetitive rhythm, like walking or swimming laps. The steady beat of your feet on the sidewalk can soothe a distracted mind or thump life into a deadened heart. Rhythmic exercise has some of the same qualities as tribal drumming: it can trance you out and subtly make your breathing become deep and regular. Best of all, you don't have to worry about scoring goals or getting hit in the teeth with a baseball. All you have to do is set your arms and legs on autopilot and forge ahead. One of many studies on the correlation between walking and mood, a 2005 study conducted at California State University found that a higher number of steps taken per day correlated positively with increased mood and energy levels.[2] Swimming has also been shown to elevate mood. No real surprises here; just get out and do it.

I could go on and weigh the benefits of various forms of exercise—indoor, outdoor, group, solo, one fish, two fish, red fish, blue fish—but you can figure that out on your own. Besides stimulating good things in your body, the simple act of exercising can make you feel organized, disciplined, competent, smarter, and more attractive. When it comes down to it, a chart of the benefits of different types of exercise would look something like this:

	Gets you fit	Makes you happy	Attracts babes
Walking	X	X	X
Jogging	X	X	X
Capoeira	X	X	X
Yoga	X	X	X
Basketball	X	X	X
Cricket	?	X?	?

Basically, exercise is a good idea. The only time it's not is if you're a compulsive exerciser or if you're too crazy to do it safely. When I lived in Vancouver, one of my favorite activities when hypomanic was to bike over the Burrard Street bridge with my eyes closed. Hot tip: bad way to get your cardio. Call a friend and do

---

2 Thayer, Robert E., et al. "Amount of Daily Walking Predicts Energy, Mood, Personality, and Health." California State University, Long Beach. Presented to American Psychological Association, 2005.

> **Instructions for Putting on Your Shoes**
> 1. Keep your shoes in a prominent place where you can find them easily (e.g., a neon pedestal at eye level marked "Shoes." It's like food in a grocery store: if your walking shoes are in a ubiquitous location, you'll be more inclined to grab them.
> 2. Pick up shoe A, stick it on your foot, and tie the laces. Repeat with shoe B. Better yet, save yourself twenty minutes and get Velcro shoes like mine.
> 3. Congratulations, you're wearing your shoes. Proceed to the next set of instructions, for leaving the house.

> **Instructions for Leaving the House**
> 1. Keep your front door in a place where you can find it easily (e.g., at the front of the house or apartment). It's like food in a grocery store: if your front door is in a ubiquitous location, you'll be more inclined to walk out of it.
> 2. If the door is locked, unlock it. You can lock it again behind you if so inclined.
> 3. Turn the doorknob. Open door.
> 4. Close door behind you if so inclined.
> 5. Congratulations, you've left the house.

something that won't result in your ass getting smeared across the front of the 22 bus.

EXERCISE FOR PEOPLE WHO HATE EXERCISE

Are you too depressed to sink a balled-up Kleenex into the trash can, let alone make a free throw? Is the farthest distance you've ever walked from your front door to a waiting taxicab when you're on your way to the club for gin and tonics? There is hope. With a little advance planning you can trick, cajole, or bitch slap yourself into at least going for a walk once a day. The key is to make it as easy and appealing as possible for yourself to get out the door, while preempting any objections or excuses you might cook up for not doing so. Remember, you're the manager, and your resistance is the slacking employee. Your job is to help yourself. Exercise isn't a punishment—it's a joy. Nine point nine times out of ten it will make you feel better *instantly*. Hold on to that thought as you spend twenty minutes tying your shoelaces.

Speaking of shoelaces, here's an interesting thought. The hardest part of getting exercise for most people is simply putting their shoes on and getting out the door. These somehow exhausting first steps trip up even the best of intentions. To help you out, here are some handy instructions you can copy and paste somewhere prominent.

In all seriousness: learn how to grit your teeth and do the above even when you don't think you feel like it. Talk yourself through the steps in a kind, gentle inner voice like Granny's: "All right sweetie, now just put your shoes on. OK now walk outside. . . ." Your *body* feels like it. Your *manager* feels like it.

Another good strategy for getting exercise is enlisting a friend. Get him/her to show up at your house every night before basketball practice so you can go together. Sign up for an aerobics class together. You don't want your friend to have to sweat her ass off *alone*, do you? If you're the type that operates best under duress, make a deal where you have to pay your friend five bucks for every sweat session you skip out on. If you're the type that responds well to bribes, route your daily walk so it goes past the bakery. Have a bank of familiar walking routes in your mind *before* it's time to go for a walk, so you're not overwhelmed with despair at not knowing where to go. That way, when you *really* don't feel like walking, it's much easier to kick yourself out the door and automatically set off on one of your preset routes. My favorite preset walk in San Francisco is to the Safeway in the Castro neighborhood. Not only is it a lovely walk with interesting buildings to look at, but also something weird always seems to be happening at that Safeway, and no matter how depressed I am, I always get a kick out of it. Last time I was there I watched a three-foot-high man with a mohawk spend twenty minutes on his cell phone with his wife debating the merits of various brands of sleepy-time tea.

Last note: If you join a gym, make sure you do it in a state of mind when you're responsible enough to make an informed financial decision. Gyms can be expensive, and trying to weasel your way out of a two-year contract you signed when you were manic is a pain in the ass. Gym memberships are like tattoos: easy to get, but friggin' impossible to get rid of.

NUTRITION, NUTRITION!

OK. Time for trusty old analogies. You have a jar. You have a pile of rocks and a pile of gravel. You want to get both the rocks and the gravel into the jar. If you put the gravel in first, the jar fills up, and there's not enough room left for all the rocks. But if you put the rocks in first, there's always room for the gravel; it trickles down to fill the spaces between the rocks.

Feeding yourself properly is like putting the rocks and gravel into the jar. The rocks are the big, essential building blocks of a healthy diet: proteins, minerals, amino acids, vitamins, good fats, and complex carbohydrates. The gravel is the stuff you want to eat outside of all that: candy, alcohol, bubble tea. The jar is your large intestine. Now there's a lot of debate over what is the number-one healthiest diet, but good nutrition comes down to this: you gotta take care of the rocks before you pour in the gravel. As a person with bipolar disorder, you're free to eat sugar and french fries like everyone else—as long as you take care of your needs for ample fresh fruits, vegetables, proteins, fats, and carbs *first*. Good nutrition isn't about cutting stuff out; it's about getting an abundance of the important stuff before throwing in the extras. Put the rocks in the jar before the gravel. But don't eat rocks—you've got bipolar disorder, not geophagia. (Unless you have bipolar disorder *and* geophagia. Talk about comorbidity!)

Whether you're a hard-core carnivore or live on Powerbars, it's in your best interest to take a look at your diet and see if there's anything you could be doing to give yourself a boost—or if there's anything you're already doing that could be aggravating your mood disorder. Make a list of everything you eat and drink in a week and compare it to the national guidelines on healthy eating. Are you getting your five to ten fruits and vegetables a day? Drinking lots of water? Living on caffeine and Tic-Tacs? Even if you think you have good eating habits, it's not a bad idea to review them for potential areas of improvement. I consider myself an extremely healthy eater, but when I stop to think about it, the only green thing I ate this week was a lime popsicle. Don't tell my mom.

Bipolar disorder is a fabulous excuse for experimenting with things like veganism or macrobiotics, treating yourself to higher-quality food, and cutting down on cheap processed stuff. You can also do a great deal of good by eating proven "mood foods" and foods you simply believe have a stabilizing effect on your mood. Here is a quick rundown of things to look out for when planning your diet.

SUGAR AND PROCESSED FOODS

Some nutritionists believe that processed foods with lots of white flour and sugar aggravate mood disorders by causing spikes in insulin that later result in blood-sugar crashes. Sugar high, sugar low. You don't need to go on a sugar witch hunt (no more ketchup! no more raisins!), but remember that too much sugar falls squarely into the gravel category, and some people find it makes bipolar symptoms worse.

FAKE SUGAR

Artificial sweeteners have gotten a bad rap for causing everything from cancer to birth defects to epilepsy. An oft-quoted study on Aspartame and depression from the *Journal of Biological Psychology* concludes, "Individuals with mood disorders are particularly sensitive to this artificial sweetener and its use in this population should be discouraged."[3] Of course, the websites for Nutra-Sweet and Aspartame deny these claims. Whether you believe the hype or not, you should at least think about how you felt the last time you drank a Diet Dr. Pepper, and if the answer is *fugly*, make future decisions accordingly.

CAFFEINE

Caffeine—friend or foe? Like many things, it's a bit of both. If you're on a high dose of something like Seroquel, you might need a cup of coffee to bust you out of your morning sleep hangover. If you're manic or getting there, the last thing you need are the wings hawked by Red Bull; chances are you've got a pair already. The link between caffeine and depression is unclear; all that is really known is that too much caffeine can contribute to insomnia, which can worsen depression (or mania). If you think getting off caffeine will help you, by all means give it a shot. Some people swear getting off caffeine and sugar was their silver bullet to health and stability. Worth a try.

OMEGA-3 FATTY ACIDS

Omega-3 fatty acids are the hot new cure for mood disorders, as vouched for by books like *The Ultimate Omega-3 Diet* that promote lots of oily fish and flaxseeds. The theory is that the human diet used to be naturally

---

3 Walton, R. "Adverse Reactions to Aspartame: Double-Blind Challenge in Patients from a Vulnerable Population." *Journal of Biological Psychology* 34(1-2), July 1–15, 1993.

rich in omega-3s until we started replacing them with omega-6s as we moved to a diet of mass-produced processed foods. This mass change in diet resulted in an increase in depression and other mental illnesses. A landmark study at Harvard University found that bipolar subjects who took about ten grams a day of omega-3 fish oil capsules experienced marked reduction in episodes of mania and depression.[4] Foods high in omega-3s include walnuts, flaxseeds, and coldwater fish like mackerel and herring. You can also buy capsules of fish or flax oil at most grocery stores and drugstores. Even if you don't believe omega-3s will help your bipolar disorder as some people claim, the evidence that they have other benefits is stacking up. Besides, fish is brain food. Try it if you feel like it. Might help.

MOOD FOODS

You've definitely seen those headlines on magazine covers in the grocery store lineup: "10 Foods That Beat Stress," "6 Foods That Make You Smarter," "99 Foods That Make You Feel Pretty Much The Same As You Felt Before." Let's face it: eating a bowl of oatmeal isn't the same thing as popping an Ativan, just like sugar isn't really the same as crack cocaine (despite what your mom says). But there's some truth to the claim that certain foods can help you calm down. The reason certain foods have calming or mood-elevating effects is because they smooth out blood-sugar levels, affect the production

---

4 Stoll, A., et al. "Omega 3 Fatty Acids in Bipolar Disorder: A Preliminary Double-Blind, Placebo-Controlled Trial." *Arch Gen Psychiatry* 56(5), May 1999.

or release of neurotransmitters, or promote serotonin production. Try incorporating some of the following into your diet.

Blood-Sugar Regulators
- oatmeal (the old-fashioned kind, not the kind loaded with sugar)
- sweet potatoes
- brown rice

Serotonin Boosters
- bananas
- salmon
- cottage cheese

Omega-3s
- flaxseeds
- salmon
- walnuts

FOOD: EAT IT ON TIME!

When you're manic or depressed, regular meals can be the first thing to fly out the window (right before your shoes, pet cactus, and roommate's bowling trophy). When I'm depressed, I often forget to eat and am always startled at how much better I feel when I finally do eat—so now I really try to monitor myself. Even when you're not manic or depressed, you can really do yourself a favor by eating several small meals spaced four to five hours apart. This keeps your blood sugar stable throughout the day, and also gives you something to look forward to every few hours. If several small meals are too much bother, stick to three meals a day, but try to eat them at the same time every day. Little routines like this are king for keeping yourself on track. Think back to Bob's Taco Shack. Bob wants his tacos delivered on time. As the manager of your own personal Taco Shack of the mind, you'd better deliver the goods to *yourself* on a consistent basis to keep things running smoothly.

FOOD: EAT IT WITH PEOPLE!

A while ago my boyfriend and I were at his parents' house for dinner. When we were driving home after the meal, he inquired about how his normally fastidious girlfriend felt about eating cheesy lasagna and cherry pie. I thought back to the dinner table. There was plenty of laughter and togetherness, and the food was home-made. Then I told him, "Eating lasagna with friends in a loving environment is healthier than eating carrot sticks alone." Not that I'd want to eat it every night. But just as exercise benefits more than your thighs, eating is about more than filling up your tank. As I'll discuss later, the social rhythm of your life can benefit you as much as your food, so double up on the goodness by sitting down to eat with people you like.

TO SLEEP, PERCHANCE TO SLEEP SOME MORE

Straight up: sleep can make or break you. Even a slight reduction in how much sleep you get can push you into a manic or depressive episode; as we've discussed, reduced sleep is both a trigger for and symptom of mania and hypomania, and insomnia is also an unfortunate feature of depression. It can't be stressed enough: get plenty of sleep, and get it around the same time each night. People with bipolar disorder are often prescribed drugs specifically for sleep, like Ambien, or drugs that make you sleepy in addition to their antipsychotic properties, like Seroquel. Whereas skipping a soccer practice won't hurtle you into dysfunction, missing a night of sleep can and will. So do whatever it takes to get yourself to bed on time, and get good sleep once you're there.

HOW TO GO TO BED

Just like you would set an alarm clock to wake you up in the morning, set yourself a literal or imaginary alarm clock to go off an hour before your target bedtime. That way, you'll have an hour to wrap up whatever you're doing and start getting into a sleepy mindset. Use visual and sensory cues to trigger your brain into sleep mode: dim the lights, light a stick of incense, clear the crap off your bed and make it up nicely so it's inviting. Make your bed a sanctuary of comfort and relaxation, not a nasty cave filled with broken potato chips and condom wrappers. If there's noise in another room, try putting on some quiet music to mask the sound. Wear earplugs and a sleeping mask. Turn off your cell phone so your raver friend Alex doesn't wake you up at 4 a.m. wondering if you want to get a burrito.

DEALING WITH INSOMNIA

If you have persistent insomnia, tell your doctor. There are tons of medications out there that are awesome for sleep, and you should be able to find one that works for you. The following advice is for the kind of insomnia you get after a hectic day at work, not the haven't-slept-in-days variety, although one can lead to the other. A big problem with insomnia is that once you've had it for one night, you spend the next day worrying about whether or not you're going to be able to fall asleep. Like a person with anorexia fretting over her next celery stick, you obsessively plan out your next sleep until the prospect of spending another night awake is so daunting you can't think of anything else.

The keys to dealing with insomnia are attitude and advance planning.

Attitude: "So what if I can't fall asleep? I'm perfectly safe, and everything's fine. I can read this book *alllll* night."

Advance Planning: Have a plan for what to do if you can't sleep. Go to a different room with soft lighting and make yourself a cup of sleepy-time tea even if you think it doesn't do anything. Have a good book to read. Try not to watch TV or use the computer, because they'll only aggravate your insomnia. Make yourself as comfortable as possible and talk yourself through it: "It's OK, I'm just going to read for a while, and whatever happens, happens." Don't fret about the fact that you can't sleep.

If you're wound up over the events of the day, write down every single worry you can think of on a piece of paper. The process of writing down the things you have to deal with gives you a sense of control and removes any fear you might have that you'll forget to do something, like send in that insurance form tomorrow. Don't pressure yourself into trying to sleep again right away. Your only job right now is to chill on the couch until you're ready to hit the sack again.

DREAMING

A weird effect of insomnia is that if you're not sleeping, you're not dreaming. And going for a while without dreaming can make you feel loss. After my first good night's sleep on medication after a long stretch without sleep, I woke up with this feeling of a lost part of myself flooding back in, and realized I'd spent all night dreaming the dreams that had been lost when I'd been trapped awake. I'm not about to venture into New Age territory here, but scientists have agreed that dreaming is pretty damn important to things like memory, and there have been reports that people with bipolar disorder experience more vivid dreams.

THIS IS YOUR MANAGER SPEAKING

Last words on self-management: be nice to your employee. Take yourself out for a milk shake now and then and listen to how things are going. Discuss franchise opportunities. Drop a quarter in the tip jar. Make awkward sexual advances in the break room. Managing yourself can be hard work, but it's worth it. Be your own best resource, make sure you get good eats, good sleeps, and good exercise, and as the fortune cookie says, you'll enjoy bountiful wealth and happiness for ten thousand moons. Ten thousand moons!

SELF-CARE Q&A

"CAN'T I JUST TAKE MY MEDS?"

"Why do I have to manage all this eating, sleeping, and exercising business? Can't I just take my meds and get on with my regular life?"

Yes, you could. But you wouldn't be doing yourself any favors. The purpose of meds is to deal with the part of your brain that is too crazy for you to manage on your own. But there's a whole lotta brain left over that you can and should manage by yourself, by establishing useful habits. Taking meds without also managing your sleep, food, and exercise is like putting on a helmet without buckling the strap under your chin, or throwing a rosary over your rearview mirror before driving drunk. You'll drastically limit the effectiveness of your medication if you don't follow through with lifestyle adaptations. And you'll drastically improve your quality of life if you *do!*

"SO I CAN'T HAVE FUN ANYMORE?"

"Yeah, right. So you're saying I have to become a raw vegan teetotaler who goes to bed at 8 p.m. You want me to have all these rules and walls around my life, man."

No offense to raw vegan teetotalers, but that's not the kind of self-management I'm advocating here. You don't have to give up partying, or your favorite foods, or your pet pony. Just take care of yourself, OK? The goal is to maximize your enjoyment of life by being as healthy, well rested, and stable as possible. Besides, what's so fun about being hospitalized or scaring away your friends anyway?

Think of it this way: You're playing a game of tennis on a court at the top of a hill. If there's no fence around the court, you technically have more freedom—freedom to spend all your time running after the ball when it bounces down the hill and into the woods. Maybe you see interesting things when you're running after the ball. Maybe these things make you a genius. Maybe they don't. If you put a fence around the tennis court, you don't have to wear yourself out chasing the ball down the hill, and you can relax and enjoy the game. Now and then the ball is still going to bounce over the fence, but it's less likely to.

How tall you make your fence depends on you. Maybe you could make yourself a short fence that allows for maximum ball escapage. Maybe build a fence so tall it's more like a cage. Either way, you end up with more court time and fewer poison ivy rashes.

6

GRACE UNDER FIRE
KEEPING A COOL HEAD IN CRAPPY SITUATIONS

If you get all flustered and freaked out every time you get depressed, or have insomnia, or overhear someone making an ignorant asshole comment about mental illness, you're going to have a long, exhausting life ahead of you. Some things are going to come up again and again over the course of your life—events that persistently trigger manic or depressive episodes; situations that make it hard to stick to your treatment plan; people who give bad or misguided advice; stupid rules, laws, and systems; traffic tickets—and you'll be much happier if you can learn to face them with grace. Instead of getting angry, scared, or belligerent every time you experience a setback, flex your grace muscle and rise to the occasion. Develop an attitude of peace and wisdom, and you'll be able to face anything that bipolar disorder throws your way.

If you observe yourself for long enough, you'll start to realize that certain things push your buttons. Winter's dark skies inevitably prompt depression, playing with ferrets makes you hypomanic, and you can't hang out with your alcoholic mother for longer than forty-five minutes without becoming full-blown psychotic. But given the way the world works, there's probably no way you can avoid winter, ferrets, or your mother for the rest of your life. So how do you deal with them?

The first step is to identify what triggers you. What were you doing and feeling in the weeks before your first manic episode? What events were going on in your life before you got depressed?

All of the following are examples of things that can trigger mania, hypomania, and depression:

- family gatherings
- exams at school
- lack of sleep
- seasons changing
- losing a job
- taking a new medication
- getting a new job
- traveling to a new time zone
- caffeine, alcohol, or drugs
- starting an exciting new project
- breaking up with someone
- starting to date someone new
- a death in the family

- traumatic events, like car crashes
- ongoing stress, like house hunting
- engaging in too much social interaction; having no time for yourself
- being too busy
- disruption to regular schedule
- new responsibility, like having a kid
- change of environment, like moving to a new apartment
- new people coming into your life

Once you have an idea of what kinds of things set you off, the next step is figuring out how to manage them happily—not necessarily avoid them or cut them out of your life. You'll have to think this through on your own. Try writing it down. For example:

Winter
- start using a light for seasonal affective disorder (SAD) in the morning.
- keep blooming plants inside (a taste of spring!)
- learn to ski (so I can maybe start loving winter)

Ferrets
- play with no more than three ferrets at a time
- limit ferret-playing time to half an hour a day
- always do a calming activity after playing with ferrets

Alcoholic Mom
- bring a friend or sibling along when I visit Mom so I'm not alone with her
- don't meet Mom in a bar (or at her house, or in her car)
- relieve stress by singing along to gangsta rap after hanging out with Mom

Don't become fearful or aversive of your triggers. Life's going to hand you what it hands you. You can't control external circumstances, but you can always adopt a proactive, graceful attitude towards whatever comes your way. You can waste a lot of time and energy stressing out about the things that make you go nuts. It's better to put that energy towards preparing a solid plan for managing them.

FACING PEOPLE

Other people are tons of fun. They want you to take their advice, date them, listen to their ideas, let them psychoanalyze you, and take body shots off their disgusting hairy chests. Other people can unwittingly say stupid things or invite you to do something that, for the sake of your health, you'd rather not do. At times people want you to eat when you're full, stay up when you'd rather sleep, drink when you'd rather be sober, and accept their (undoubtedly brilliant and insightful) analysis of your moods when you know they're full of hot air. Learn how to assert your will, conclusively yet without sounding like a jerk. Only you know what you need, and only you can assert yourself.

TEN WAYS YOU CAN TACTFULLY SAY NO TO SOMETHING
"Nah, I'm taking it easy tonight."

"Healing crystals worked for your aunt? That's interesting."

"Dude, if I have another cup of coffee, I'm going to climb the walls!"

"Yo, being angry isn't the same thing as being bipolar."

"I'm gonna hit the sack, guys. Goodnight."

"Going off meds worked for your mailman? Fascinating. Tell me again about his rifle collection."

"No thanks, I'm so over doing cocaine off toilet tanks."

"I'm not drunk. I'm just happy 'cause it's my birthday!"

"Dude, I really don't think your boss is bipolar."

"Need to get my beauty rest. See y'all in the morning."

Sometimes, other people can be really smart. They have good suggestions, insightful observations, and make well-meaning offers. But the same defense mechanisms we erect against bad suggestions can also keep out good ones. We reject perfectly good, heartfelt offers out of sheepishness, embarrassment, and irritability. To rephrase the AA prayer: "Lord, give me the grace to reject the suggestions that really suck, to accept the ones that don't, and the wisdom to know the difference."

TEN WAYS YOU CAN SAY YES TO SOMETHING WITHOUT LOSING FACE

"You're right, I have been a little short on sleep lately."

"Sure, I'd love to borrow your book about binaural beats."

"Yeah, I would like it if you came over tonight."

"Hey, pass it to the left!"

"You know what, I never saw it that way before."

"I changed my mind. I'd love to have dinner with you guys."

"A SAD light helped your brother? That's so interesting!"

"Let's go for that walk after all."

"Yeah, I'm just drinking orange juice tonight. Cheers!"

"Man, I'm really not making sense today, am I?"

Always remember that you have more choices than you think you have about how to deal with a stressful situation. Which options are you overlooking? What are your alternatives to reacting negatively? How can you subtly manage your reactions to turn the situation into a learning experience rather than a trigger?

FACING DEPRESSION

The best tool I've learned for overcoming depression is one that my doctor and psychiatrist never mentioned. It's a game. My boyfriend showed it to me, and we play it whenever I get depressed. It goes like this:

He says, "How long have you been sad?" and I invariably wail, "Forever!" Then we sit down together and recall happy events. He says, "I remember how we went jogging in Mexican wrestler masks last week and that little kid and his dad chased us down the street." I sniff and gulp, "That was pretty fun." He says, "And remember how you put on reggae music and danced around in a sheet to wake me up the other morning?" I nod and say, "It was so nice and sunny that day." Soon enough, I start adding happy memories to our list and start remembering that life isn't all a crushing, futile disaster.

Recalling happy memories is a massage for your brain. It stimulates the production of happy chemicals similar to the chemicals produced when you were actually experiencing the happy event. And it helps you remember that you're not an inherently grieving, sorrowful person; your baseline mood is actually quite happy, and as soon as this depression is over with you'll be back those feelings of happiness. Another term for baseline mood is "hedonic set point."

Your hedonic set point, often called the "happiness thermostat," is your standard level of happiness. Very cheerful people have their hedonic thermostats set on high, and more subdued people have their thermostats set a little lower. When you're not manic or depressed, your mood hovers around your hedonic set point, rising and falling a little bit in response to the day's ups and downs, but always gravitating towards that point. When you become manic or depressed, your mood flies way above or below your hedonic set point. The goal of medication and therapy is to get you to stay within a healthy range of your hedonic set point, rather than swinging way out of bounds.

Playing the remembering game is a great way of resetting your brain to its natural hedonic set point. It's a beautiful, natural, and completely free form of therapy that really works. (Curiously, if you do it enough, research shows its one of the few things that actually *raises* your hedonic set point—better than therapists, books, and almost everything else except meds.)

FACING YOURSELF AFTER MANIA OR HYPOMANIA

Manic and hypomanic episodes can be fun or exciting, but the fun stops when the episode's over. Then, as the smoke clears and you start to remember what you got up to during the episode, the exhilaration is all too often replaced with embarrassment, regret, and shame: "Oh shit . . . I really did make out with that forty-year-old stranger who looks like a hedgehog, jump on a crowded bus and loudly recite Yeats for the whole ride home, and chop the living room couch in half with an axe. What will my roommates think?"

The most important thing to remind yourself in this situation is that you didn't do whatever you did because you're inherently slutty or arrogant or violent—you're struggling with a serious disorder. Should your friend who has the flu be embarrassed for throwing up in your sink? You happen to have mania—sprees and flights of fancy are symptoms, just like vomiting is a symptom of influenza. If you're feeling bad about something you said or did to another person while manic or hypomanic, it's totally cool to call that person up and say, "Hey, I didn't mean it when I said . . ." or "I'm really sorry I broke your chair while I was manic. Can I fix it?" Most friends who know about your bipolar disorder will just be relieved to hear you're feeling better. And for friends who don't know about your bipolar disorder, this is an opportune time to have a conversation about it.

There's no point lingering on the things you did while you were manic, because you can't go back and change them. All you can do is work on having a good day *today*, and plan how to take care of yourself super-well so you can avoid having another manic episode next week.

FACING INSOMNIA

Insomnia curses millions of people every night. And if you curse back, it only gets harder to sleep. It's a slippery slope: you couldn't sleep last night, so you worry about whether you'll be able to sleep tonight, and that makes sleeping impossible. Your mind lit up by worry, you unwittingly turn yourself into a sleep-proof vessel. Sleep couldn't break through to you if it *tried*. Hours spent awake when you'd rather be sleeping are torture; you're not doing something productive, but you're not resting either. You're trapped in limbo, useless as a broken lightbulb.

To make insomnia more bearable and get over it faster, learn to weather it peacefully. Instead of "Goddamn it, why can't I sleep?" think "Ah, I'm awake. Let's see how I can make myself comfortable." Getting insomnia is like getting a parrot when you were expecting a kitten: it's not what you wanted, but since you have it, you might as well be nice to it and teach it cool tricks. Making the parrot angry won't help matters (angry parrots tend to attack), and getting angry at the parrot won't turn it into a kitten.

So you have insomnia. Get out of bed, make yourself a cup of herbal tea, and sit down in a quiet, lamp-lit room with a good book. Don't struggle to fix your insomnia or beat it into submission. Just be there, calm and peaceful, a good friend to yourself.

Repeat as many nights as necessary.

FACING STIGMA

A little while ago I wanted to go to a meditation retreat in the foothills of Yosemite National Park. The website for the retreat claimed that everybody in the world could benefit from the universal truths of this meditation technique. But a little further down, it stated that people with bipolar disorder and schizophrenia were forbidden from attending the retreat.

Even the most enlightened people can be guilty of stigmatizing.

A stigma comes from the false belief that a person is unable to perform certain tasks or achieve certain heights, by virtue of belonging to a stigmatized category. Instead of looking at an individual's talents and abilities, a stigma says, "You belong to category bipolar; therefore, you must have qualities x and y that make you unfit to meditate/get health insurance/get a promotion/become president." People use stigmas to justify treating other people unfairly.

Don't let the ignorance other people carry in their hearts hurt you. Stand up to stigmas by staying calm and demonstrating through reason and example the fallacy of the stigmatic belief. If you just say, "Screw you," you give people the power to keep looking down on you. If you keep your head, you have a better chance of showing them up for how wrong they are. Don't get mad—get even.

P.S. I got even by attending that meditation retreat anyway. (It was free.) Guess what? Having bipolar disorder didn't have any effect on my ability to meditate. Funny thing.

FACING DISAPPOINTMENT

Unless you're a rapid cycler, you're going to have periods of time between manic and depressive episodes when you just feel happy and normal. Having an episode after a long period of happiness and normality can be crushingly disappointing. When you're stable for long enough—months or years—you naturally start to forget a little about what it feels like to be manic or depressed. Those parts of your life are all in the past. You feel confident that you can remain stable indefinitely. Though you would never express it out loud, you secretly feel like you're finished with bipolar. You're over it, you've grown out of it, you've cracked the code to staying well.

Then it suddenly happens again—the depressive slop, the manic fire. All the foundations you laid so well start to crumble, and you find yourself feeling emotions you thought you were done with forever. You feel terrible shame for your cockiness at thinking you had risen above bipolar, and you feel guilt too, because you perceive that you've let down your family, significant other, and psychiatrist (repeat after me: billable hours) for becoming manic or depressed again.

The truth is, the nature of bipolar disorder is to cycle back again and again. We can take medication to slow down the cycles and reduce their severity, and we can practice good self-management for the same reason. But as yet there's no way to permanently stop future episodes from happening.

Think of an apple tree that changes throughout the seasons. Do you get angry at an apple tree and chop it down when it loses its leaves in the winter and seems to die? No—you wait for spring, when it will flower and bear fruit again. You can't stop the seasons from changing. You're not shocked and appalled when summer turns to fall. Why should the changing seasons of your mood be a source of distress?

Nothing's permanent. You'll never be permanently stable, or (God help you) permanently depressed or manic, or permanently young, or permanently in love with your tongue ring. Though, I will confess, that snake-eating-a-unicorn tattoo still does look pretty sweet. Meet all your changing seasons with love.

7

HERE BE DOWNERS
DRUGS, BOOZE, AND SUICIDE

One of the biggest downers of being diagnosed bipolar is getting slapped with a ton of statistics. Your parents read a book about bipolar, and suddenly everyone's breathing down your neck about your newfound Risk of Suicide! Risk of Alcoholism! Risk of Drug Abuse! Risk of Speeding on the Freeway! Risk of Taking Lots of Risky Risks!

It's true that people with bipolar disorder have a higher than average tendency to have problems with drugs and alcohol and make suicide attempts. The former tends to play into the latter. Mania, alcohol, and drugs can all lower your inhibitions and make you more likely to act on a suicidal urge. And depression, especially when combined with alcohol or drugs, can get you low enough to make suicide look like a pleasant alternative to another day in the sunshine. But just because the statistics are bad doesn't mean that you, personally, will develop a problem. And if you do develop a problem with suicidal thoughts or addiction, it's not the end of the world. There are ways of coping with and overcoming these hindrances and support systems to help you along the way. Suicide, drug addiction, and alcoholism are real-life ogres lurking in the forest of bipolar disorder (and in plenty of other forests too). Looking them in the face is the first step to diminishing their power. (Side note: why can't more forests be stocked with bunnies?)

SUICIDE

When you go hiking in the Rockies, there are posters at the trailheads telling you what to do if you encounter a grizzly bear. I always read these posters avidly, because as a frequent hiker I would really, really like some solid instructions on what to do if this happened to me. Yet time after time I'm frustrated: the instructions are always vague, saying things like "stay calm" and "leave the area." Leave the area? What if there's another bear behind me? I've questioned rangers about this, and after reciting the usual Grizzly Bear Protocol, they shrug and say, "You just have to think on your feet."

Feeling suicidal is like having a grizzly bear encounter. Everybody has some general idea of what you should do if you feel suicidal ("leave the area!"), but when you get down to specific variables ("But what if there are *two* bears?"), it becomes obvious that nobody has a fucking clue. It's a scary, high-stakes, high-risk situation, and you're just gonna have to work with whatever you can grab (which is hopefully a telephone or your best friend's hand).

The stats on bipolar and suicide are terrible (and wildly variant). The quotes are all over the map. You can find stats claiming that anywhere from 10 to 50 percent of people with bipolar disorder attempt suicide. Seriously, guys? Fifty percent? Then you find out that their test pool consisted of a thousand recently bankrupt, grief-stricken, rapid-cycling sixty-year-olds on their fortieth hospitalization. Maybe *that* test pool has a 50 percent likelihood of attempting suicide. Attempting—not even completing. Another test pool might have a 20 percent likelihood of attempting suicide. For another test pool, it might be 15 percent.

Don't trust statistics. Statistics know nothing about you. That being said, having bipolar disorder does place you at a higher risk of suicide than the general population, and there are certain factors within bipolar that can place you at an even higher risk. I've decided to edit out the numbers ("eating pudding makes you two point twelve times as likely") because the whole point of this book is to make you feel less like a human scorecard and more like a human. But here are the risk factors themselves:

- *Frequency of hospitalization*
  The biggest factor associated with suicide attempts among people with bipolar disorder is being hospitalized several times. If you've been in and out of hospital several times, you're more likely to attempt suicide at some point. This is why it's important to take all the measures you can to stay stable (especially by taking meds and living right)—so that you can go through the psychiatric wringer as few times as humanly possible.
- *Depressive or mixed first episode*
  If your first episode was depressive or mixed, your risk of attempting suicide is higher than if your first episode was manic or hypomanic.

- *Stressful life events before the onset of bipolar disorder*

  If the onset of your bipolar disorder was precipitated by a gnarly life event, like physical abuse, you have a higher risk of attempting suicide.

- *Episodes occurring without downtime in between*

  If you have episode after episode after episode with no symptom-free intervals in between, then—you guessed it!—you have a higher risk of attempting suicide. That psychiatric wringer can wear a person out pretty fast.

- *Drug and alcohol abuse*

  Don't abuse drugs and alcohol, kids. It raises your risk of acting on impulses, which raises your risk of attempting suicide.

- *Family history*

  If you have bipolar disorder *and* a family member who committed suicide, your risk of attempting suicide is higher than the general population. It's like alcoholism: if your parents were alcoholics, you're genetically at risk for developing alcoholism yourself.

It seems logical that you can reduce your risk of suicide by going through the list of risk factors and minimizing the ones it's within your power to minimize. But insofar as people commit suicide in response to stressful life events, the only way you can really protect yourself is by developing sound strategies for dealing with stress, grief, and suicidal thoughts—or by sealing yourself in a bubble. And insofar as suicide is a symptom of bipolar disorder, the best way to protect yourself is to take measures to stay stable and have as few episodes as possible, so that this terrible symptom doesn't get too many chances to rear its ugly head.

The first thing you should do if you have suicidal thoughts (doctors call this "ideation") is to talk to your psychiatrist. Suicidal thoughts are sometimes a side effect of psychiatric drugs, and you might need a change in your medications. And if your suicidal thoughts *aren't* a side effect, that's all the more reason to get help immediately. Don't be embarrassed or squeamish. If the brakes on your car stopped working, you wouldn't sit around dithering whether they're broken *enough* to warrant a check-in with the mechanic. Ditto thoughts of suicide.

If you feel actively suicidal (i.e., imminently about to kill yourself), holler at everyone you possibly can and ask them for help. Get on the crisis telephone line and talk to a counselor (1-800-273-TALK), call your psychiatrist if you have one, and get your mom or uncle or best friend or neighbor to drive over and pick you up. You can even go to the emergency room or call 911. There is an unbelievably huge and passionate and loving suicide-prevention community out there; they care about you, and it would make their friggin' day to save your life. So please let them.

The most important things when you're feeling suicidal are to: (a) call people who can help you and (b) not be alone. Whatever you do, don't start drinking or taking drugs to help you deal with your suicidal thoughts, because these things will only make you more likely to act on them. It's a good idea to keep a list of emergency phone numbers in your wallet or in your cell phone contacts list so you don't need to scramble to find them when it's down to the wire. Remember that suicidal thoughts are a symptom of your disorder; they are not real, normal thoughts. Feeling suicidal is like having a heart attack or running into a grizzly bear when you're hiking: it's not your fault; it's just something that's *out there*.

ONE WAY OF UNDERSTANDING SUICIDAL THOUGHTS
Think of it this way.

Suicidal thoughts are a symptom of bipolar. Bipolar is a medical condition, like having a cold, and the symptoms of bipolar are like coughs and a runny nose. Even though it feels more intimate and personal, suicidal ideation is just as impersonal as chills and a fever. When the episode clears up, it clears up (and if it doesn't, you should tell your psychiatrist). Suicidal thoughts can be very scary, and if you think of them this way—as a symptom, as a trick your mind is playing on you as part of a disease— you can place them in a less scary context.

When I was really depressed in Vancouver, I had recurring thoughts of filling my backpack with rocks, taking a lot of Seroquel, and jumping off the Burrard Street Bridge. I think the logic was that I would be too sleepy to notice I was drowning. What helped me get through that time was understanding those thoughts metaphorically—as a painful, hacking cough that was a completely impersonal symptom of depression, nothing more. People who meditate love this stuff; they call it detachment. The thinking goes that you can peacefully observe negative thoughts and sensations without making them personal, and by not getting involved with them, you don't get hurt by them.

Old thought: "I'm so depressed. This grief is unbearable. Every moment is a living death. I want to die."

Detached thought: "Ah, it appears I am experiencing grief! Hello, grief. It appears I am having thoughts of suicide! Hello, thoughts of suicide."

By practicing this kind of thinking, you can help yourself disarm the power of suicidal thoughts and other negative emotions—at least enough to survive until you're able to get further help. You establish that *you* are not the same thing as your thoughts, and you not subject to suffering from them. It takes practice and isn't a replacement for medication or the support of a doctor (until you become a fully enlightened being, that is), but it can do you lots of good. Practicing detachment helps you realize that your pain isn't permanent, and you, therefore, don't need the permanent solution of suicide to get rid of it.

MORE ABOUT SUICIDE

When somebody commits suicide, it's upsetting not only because of the grief of losing that person, but also because suicide makes us realize how fragile life is—and that each of us has the stunning power to take our own life. Anybody old enough to walk has the power to kill themselves at pretty much any time, yet, by and large, we don't. Suicide reminds us that the line between life and death is always with us, always crossable, even when we forget it's there.

Even if you never attempt suicide, having bipolar disorder can make you more aware of this fine line between life and death. Don't we take medication that drags us back from the "death" of depression? Don't we occasionally take wild, uncharacteristic risks, survive them, and realize death isn't as surefire a consequence as people think? Like running across a busy street during mania: "Wow, I can do this and not die. Am I a god? Am I invincible? Is my red sweater a charm making me immune to death?" And in depression: "How can I feel this bad and still be alive? Death must be something you experience every waking moment, not a special occasion that happens at the end of your life." For a severely depressed person, death can seem a constant, the most real and inescapable thing in the world, and for a manic person who has "cheated death," death dissolves into an abstract, unlikely joke. Maybe our ongoing flirtations with Señor Death, in addition to our weird brain chemistry, make people with bipolar more likely to actually cross the line.

"SO WHAT HAPPENS IF I ATTEMPT SUICIDE?"

Well, for starters you could die. And as much fun as that sounds, I'm not coming after you. (Actually, I will, eventually, but this is neither here nor there.)

If you don't die, you'll be found or stopped by somebody and taken to the emergency room. This is what goes down when you go to the emergency room following a suicide attempt:

The emergency-room staff stabilize you physically (by pumping your stomach, extracting the bullet from your chest, sewing up your arms, etc.) and emotionally (by sedating you). They do tests to see if you're drunk, on street drugs, or on medication that might be causing a suicidal side effect. Next, you'll go through a mental-health assessment, where they'll try to figure out how crazy you are, whether your craziness is acute or chronic, whether you have previous suicide attempts, and why you tried to commit suicide this time. You, your family, and the doctors will talk about treatment options and support systems that are available to you. Next, the emergency-department personnel will decide if you need to be hospitalized, either of your own free will or by having you committed. If they decide to have you committed, a legal process will ensue that will take from three to ten days. If they decide you don't need to be hospitalized, you'll be sent home with a plan to check in with your doctor regularly and stay away from guns and knives.

"WHAT'S IT LIKE CALLING A CRISIS TELEPHONE LINE?"

Crisis telephone lines are staffed by counselors or trained volunteers whose job it is to get you through your immediate crisis and point you towards further help. If you're calling because you feel suicidal, the person who answers will listen to you, reflect your problems back to you, and encourage you to keep talking and stay on the line. At the end of the call, she'll refer you to a service in your area, such as a drop-in crisis center or clinic you can go to.

Oh yeah, you don't have to be on the verge of suicide to call. These peeps are there for you *whenever*. You can call them to cry about breaking up with Steve. They won't hang up on you. If you don't have a psychiatrist to call, a crisis phone line is a good bet, because the act of calling is in itself a diversion from whatever destruction you're about to wreak. Check out the Resources section for crisis lines in the United States and Canada.

DRUGZ 'N' BOOZE

Tons of people with bipolar disorder self-medicate with drugs and alcohol, and this often turns into addiction that makes bipolar even harder to treat.

Why do we turn to drugs and alcohol in the first place, and why are we more prone to developing addictions? What are our reasons for using drugs and alcohol to self-medicate?

"IT'S MY BEST FRIEND'S BIRTHDAY, I'VE BEEN SEVERELY DEPRESSED FOR WEEKS, AND I JUST REALLY, REALLY WANT TO BE HAPPY TONIGHT. I'M GOING TO HAVE A DRINK OR TWO IN PRIVATE BEFORE WE GO OUT TO DINNER."

When you're depressed, it can be tempting to use alcohol as a bootstrap to get you into a happy mood. Upside: if it works, and you have a good time at your friend's birthday, you feel better about yourself—happy that you finally felt happy, and more positive about getting over your depression. Downside: lingering feelings of guilt about hiding your drinking, feeling that your friend would be let down if she knew you were tipsy at her birthday, falsely believing you've found a workable backup plan for future social events. Plus, alcohol's a depressant, affecting some of the same brain receptors as your meds, so you could be screwing up the very thing you're trying to fix. The grounds are laid for future alcohol reliance and abuse. To be fair, you could conceivably use alcohol "just this once" and never do it again, but it's a friend that tends to come sneaking back. And if you're genetically predisposed to alcoholism, then it goes without saying: here be dragons.

"IT'S THE ONLY THING THAT HELPS ME SLEEP."

When I lived in the crowded, mice-ridden staff accommodations at a hotel in Jasper, Alberta, it was noisy and bright until three in the morning, and my shift started at 6 a.m. Sometimes, the only way to get to sleep at night was to make a Quetiapine-Trazodone-Nytol cocktail and chase it with a couple swigs of white wine. After all, I thought, sleep is my one link to sanity, and if I have to tranquilize the hell out of myself to get there, so be it. This method left me feeling blurry and sick in the morning, lowered my self-esteem, and did me no favors for my job performance as the switchboard operator in charge of bright and cheerful morning wake-up calls.

It should be insanely obvious that using alcohol to get to sleep is a bad idea, and it's even stupider if you combine it with your meds. You can develop an alcohol dependence without even trying, and counter the effects of your medication in the process. There are so many options out there for good sleep—endless pharmaceuticals, as well as non-pharmaceutical techniques, like meditation—that there's no excuse for using alcohol to get to sleep (except having an alcohol problem).

"EVERYONE ELSE GETS TO PARTY. WHY CAN'T I?"

If you're the kind of person who doesn't like being told what to do, being told that drugs and alcohol are especially risky for you can make you want to party even harder. You drink and do drugs even harder than usual to prove that you're not crazy or weak, that you're still wild and fun even though you're on meds, and that you can take it like a man/woman just like everyone else.

Real power is knowing innately that you have nothing to prove. Abusing drugs and alcohol in response to a bipolar diagnosis isn't evidence that you're stronger than them; it's evidence of how much you think you need them in order to keep your self-image intact. If being yourself depends on getting drunk—such an ephemeral, external thing—then who are you? Having bipolar doesn't necessarily mean you can't drink or party anymore—plenty of bipolar people do, safely and happily. It's entirely possible for a person with bipolar who doesn't have alcoholic genes to drink without become an alcoholic, or smoke a peace pipe without becoming a pothead. But don't bring drugs and alcohol into your life in order to prove a point or self-medicate your bipolar, because it's an enterprise more futile than putting out a flaming outhouse with gasoline.

"WHAT IF I'M ALREADY ADDICTED?"

If you are living with alcoholism or a drug addiction, you need to deal with that if you ever hope to stabilize your bipolar cycles.

Alcoholism and drug addiction co-occur with bipolar an awful lot. Are more alcoholics and drug addicts bipolar, or do more people with bipolar develop alcoholism and addiction? Chicken and egg scenario? Alcoholism or addiction can make bipolar disorder nearly impossible to treat, because the drinking and drugs exacerbate your mood cycles and interfere with your medication. Plus, it's hard to tell which of your symptoms are caused by bipolar and which are from the drinking or drugs. Slapping a drug addiction or alcoholism on top of bipolar disorder is like feeding expired food to a person with the flu: they vomit twice as much, and now you can't tell if it's the virus or the botulism.

This is not an addiction- or alcoholism-recovery book. My advice? Get your ass to an Alcoholics Anonymous meeting. Help is out there, and you deserve to get it.

8

THE GAME OF LIFE
BIPOLAR IN COLLEGE AND AT WORK

Remember that Dr. Seuss book *Green Eggs and Ham,* about this creature who would eat green eggs and ham just about anywhere? Mania and depression are kind of like that—they can sneak up on you whether you're in a boat or with a goat, in the rain, on a train. You're going to have to tend to the peculiarities of your brain throughout college, travel, and jobs—and some situations take more brain-tending than others. Might as well do your best to make college and work support your bipolar disorder, not aggravate it. The game of life can work for you, if you're good at tweaking the system in your favor.

COLLEGE: A HEAVEN FOR THE MENTALLY ILL

Colleges are wonderlands of free or cheap resources that can help you get through your crazy times. Now's the time to tax those resources for all they're worth. Your college probably has a few of the following things.

- *Free gym or swimming pool for stress relief*
  A quick swim or workout between classes is especially useful if you're depressed, because exercise boosts your

energy and makes you feel good about yourself. Plus, you don't have to talk to anybody while you're doing it.

- *Free drop-in counseling*

  Some colleges have peer-counseling centers where you can drop in and talk to someone confidentially. You might feel self-conscious the first time, but remember, they're here for you—and they volunteered!

- *Free periods of extreme stress followed by periods of substance abuse and boredom*

  To keep you cycling.

- *Quiet lounges*

  My university was lounge happy. There was a women's lounge, a Native American lounge, a meditation lounge, a sustainability lounge—and most of them were massively underused. Underused lounges are the perfect place to escape from the world and grab a nap in the middle of the day, and they often have free tea and a microwave.

- *Student groups*

  Depending on the size of your university, it might have an Active Minds or Depression Bipolar Support Alliance chapter, or another group devoted to mental-health issues. A listing of good mental-health organizations can be found in the Resources section.

- *Nooks and crannies*

  Music practice rooms, library study cubicles, boat docks, and other such places offer privacy and quiet in the midst of the hectic university environment. If you need to go someplace to chill out or cry (or make out with someone), these nooks and crannies come in handy.

- *Pretty foresty stuff*

  Many university campuses have some kind of nice natural feature like a forest or pond or beach or even a garden. This makes it really convenient to catch some "green time" between classes. Hanging out with trees and plants is good for you. It can even be kind of addictive. Try it out.

- *People*

  University campuses are full of people who know or recognize you. Even if you only have two real friends, there are at least two dozen people who recognize you as "the tall guy with red shoes" and a handful of professors who know you as "guy in second row." If you're feeling lonely, hanging out on campus is a step up from being alone in your room—and you're much more likely to run into someone you know.

- *Library*

  If you're hypomanic or manic and feeling spendy, you can check out a hundred library books instead of blowing all your money. Checking out books gives you a similar rush, and as long as you return the books later, costs nothing.

- *Productivity and distraction*

  There's always something productive or distracting to do at a university. Crank out an essay, go to a free play or concert, or sit in on a class.

- *For people with mental illnesses, generous policies on dropping classes, changing schedules, or taking a term off*

  Universities are, by definition, progressive places. Don't be afraid to use bipolar as a medical reason for forcing your way into an afternoon class rather than an early morning one, taking fewer courses than usual, or fulfilling some of your graduation requirements online.

COLLEGE: A HELL FOR THE MENTALLY ILL

If you're dealing with a mental illness, college can be a torture palace. You can be isolated and lonely, despite being surrounded by people; overwhelmed by assignments and events; and worn ragged by the endless pressure and stimulation. When you juggle bipolar disorder with college, you might run into a few of the following:

- *Overwork*

  You have a lab report, a life-sized charcoal self-portrait, and a twenty-page essay due on Monday. What other option do you have but to stay awake all weekend to finish them?
- *Crappy schedule*

  Your first class is at 8 a.m., but your roommate likes to play death metal until 3 a.m. Your lunch break is from 3 to 3:30 p.m., and by that time you've been starving and distracted for hours.
- *Overstimulation*

  It never stops. You go to class, go to the gym, do some homework, go out for dinner with friends, go out for drinks, then go to a club and dance until it closes. Repeat three or four times a week.
- *Loneliness*

  You're hellishly depressed, but nobody in your dorm even notices that you haven't left your room in three days. You don't even know your professors' names, and you would be mortified to ask for an extension on a project.
- *Alcohol and/or drugs*

  Everyone parties all the time. You can't escape it—there's some kind of beer garden or house party or drunken grocery-cart racing every day of the week. It seems like you can't be at a social event that doesn't involve drinking.

BALANCING HEAVEN AND HELL AT COLLEGE

The items in the first list should help you deal with some of the items in the second list. If overwork is driving you into hypomania, drop a class. If you're not getting enough sleep, schedule afternoon or evening classes instead of morning ones. If you need less stimulation and more alone time, take one of your classes online, so you can do it without even leaving your room. If you feel isolated, join a group and go to drop-in counseling. It's especially important to support yourself in these ways if you're returning to college after a period of hospitalization. It's not easy to go back into a demanding college environment after spending six months so doped up it took you fifteen minutes to figure out how to roll the dice when you were playing Candyland with your psych ward roommate. Cut yourself some slack!

CLASSES: DROP 'EM LIKE THEY'RE HOT

If you go nuts while you're in college and don't get proper documentation of your Gone Nuts status, you can end up with a ton of failed classes and maybe even screw up your chances of graduating. So make sure you get a shrink's note stating that you were unable to attend classes/exams for health reasons, and fill out any forms your university or college dean's office requires to make it official. With a note from your shrink, you can drop a class after the official drop date, defer completing an online class for a semester or two, arrange a semester off, and defer graduating until you're healthy enough to get your work done. (Other perks: free underage booze, free strippers, and all-access backstage passes. Just bring your note to Bono and tell him your psychiatrist sent you.)

In general, dropping or deferring classes and/or graduation requires a pile of forms and signatures—usually a combination of the following items.

- Medical documentation (e.g., note from your psychiatrist)
- An add/drop form with your professor's signature
- A signature from your academic advisor
- A signature from the dean

Your school registrar's office can tell you exactly which forms and signatures you need. Chasing all these people down can be a bitch, but it's even more of a bitch *not* to do it and end up with failed classes.

ALIENATION

Coming down with a disorder that messes with your sense of reality can make you seriously reevaluate your life choices. The endless treadmill of reading and spitting out essays, memorizing equations and spitting out assignments, can feel meaningless—howlingly, grievously meaningless—when held up to the light of your experiences. Your eyes have been opened to a completely different worldview than that of most of your professors and classmates, and it can be hard to buckle down and think about geology when you just got back from the dark side if the moon, man.

Now and then bipolar disorder will make you slow down and ask yourself, am I living right? Are the things I'm pursuing really worth pursuing? Do I want what I want? Do I know what I know?

Then you forget about the big questions and slip into your old patterns, until next time.

I found that the best way to deal with alienation in college was to befriend myself and to integrate my personal insights into my academic work wherever it made sense to do so. Women's Studies class? Perfect venue to write an essay about homelessness and mental-health issues among Canadian women. Eighteenth-century literature class? Edmund Burke's theory of the sublime is fascinating to consider in the light of twenty-first-century mental-hospital narratives. If your mind is constantly grappling with the idea of being mentally ill anyway, you might as well take advantage of your academic setting to explore those ideas in detail. Take whatever you find soulless and mundane and find ways to make it meaningful. Direct your powers for good instead of evil.

BE YOUR OWN MENTAL ASYLUM

Give yourself permission to drop a class, walk out of a lecture, or take a day off school if you need to in order to stay afloat mentally. The biggest mistake you can make when you're coming back to college after a breakdown is trying to do everything at once—classes, clubs, part-time job, socializing. Take it slow—three classes a semester instead of five, a house party on the weekend instead of nightly clubbing. It's better to take it easy and graduate a semester late than overload yourself and end up in the hospital, which sets you back a year.

It helps to set aside little shelters for yourself throughout the day or week. Take yourself out for coffee and have a nice, long, regrouping conversation with yourself. Skip the bar now and then and go for a walk instead. Get away from the endless hustle of campus and spend time on the beach or in the woods. Treat yourself kindly; you've just come out of an experience that's wildly out of whack with the rest of the world, and it takes time to readjust. Don't just throw yourself to the wolves. Go gently. Do it right.

THE WORKPLACE: A HEAVEN FOR THE MENTALLY ILL

Having a job can have all sorts of beneficial effects, both hidden and not so hidden, on your mood. Unless your job totally sucks, it probably provides a few of the following:

- *Health insurance*
  Don't underestimate the value of a job that gives you health benefits. As we'll see in a later chapter, it's extremely hard to get individual insurance in the United States if you have bipolar on your rap sheet.
- *Steady schedule*
  Having a job with regular hours forces you to go to bed and get up at roughly the same time each day. This can be great for mood stability.
- *Social network*
  Even if you aren't best friends with your coworkers, having a job increases the number of people who know you and will notice if you're acting weird. Plus, if you don't show up for work, someone's bound to notice—always a good thing if you're prone to overdosing on sleeping pills.
- *Dollar billz*
  If you've been dependent on your parents your whole life, making money gives you a feeling of independence and self-determination you can't get any other way.

- *Meaning*

  Doing meaningful work is great for your health, especially if you can see that your work is having a visible effect on the world. If you're depressed, work can keep your mind off your emotions, and if you're hypomanic, work keeps you busy so you don't get into trouble (unless you get your hands on the staple gun).

THE WORKPLACE: A HELL FOR THE MENTALLY ILL

Work can totally mess with your system and exacerbate your mania or depression. The world is full of bitchy managers and bosses who don't give a crap about anything short of bribing the health and labor law inspectors. With any job, watch out for the following:

- *Overwork*

  Just like in college, you might find yourself overburdened with tasks and projects that stay on your mind well past working hours. Do they seriously think *one person* is enough to do the accounting for the entire corporation?

- *Crappy schedule*

  Your job starts at 6 a.m., but you can never get to sleep until 2 a.m. Or your schedule's constantly changing, and you can never establish a stable rhythm. Or you're on call twenty-four hours a day—so when the hell are you supposed to take your slumber-inducing antipsychotics?

- *Meaninglessness*

  Three months ago you realized you were the new messiah, but now you're stabilized and on meds and working at Blockbuster. Meaningful work? Ha! Mary Magdalene would weep tears of blood if she could see you now (or if you could see her—which you can't because you're not psychotic anymore. Shit!).

- *Social scumduggery*

  You're not best friends with your coworkers. In fact, they're the most obnoxious, vicious, ignorant gang of villains you've ever met. They have no idea where you're coming from and frequently make you cry. Oh yeah, and you're supposed to go out for drinks with them after work.

BALANCING HEAVEN AND HELL AT WORK

Not all jobs are worth salvaging. If you hate your job, quit and find a better one. If you have a job that you like, tweak it to make it a job you love—and a job that won't aggravate your bipolar disorder. If changing schedules is a problem, request to be put on the same shift every day. If you show up with a doctor's note, the employer should accommodate your request. If you work in an office, you might be able to work from home one or several days a week. No matter where you work, know your rights in regards to break times. If you're legally allowed two fifteen-minute breaks and a half-hour lunch, take them. Go for a walk, get some fresh air, have a snack, and stay sane.

SELF-EMPLOYMENT

Do you even need a traditional job? There are other ways of supporting yourself than slaving away for a boss or company that doesn't know you exist. Aren't people with bipolar more creative than usual? More resourceful than usual? More willing to take risks than usual?

If crappy jobs are a problem, why not work for yourself? You set your own schedule, choose what kind of work you take on, and develop all sorts of tasty new skills and business savvy in the process. There's no depressing office, you're nobody's bitch, and if you need to take a mental-health day, nobody can tell you otherwise.

Self-employment is a great option in the short term if you're too crazy for or can't commit to a full-time job, and a great option in the long term if you fall in love with how freeing and rewarding it is.

Some ideas:

- Teach music lessons
- Make and sell something
- Resell stuff on eBay
- Offer a service in your field of expertise
- Freelance writing
- House-sitting

If you decide to be self-employed, make sure you still get health insurance. Check out the health insurance chapter for more details on that little conundrum.

TAKING A MENTAL-HEALTH DAY

Whether you're at school, at work, or working for yourself, there are going to be days when you just need to check out of the world or you just *know* you're going to have an episode. Give yourself a break. It's way better to take a day off and let yourself cool down than to keep on working or schooling and run yourself into a manic or depressive episode. The ultimate mental-health day is the equivalent of pushing the reset button; you turn back the clock a little and let yourself unwind.

My ultimate mental-health day goes as follows:

10 a.m.: Get extra sleep, then wake up and spend time making decent breakfast (oatmeal with walnuts and fruit—good for the brain!).

10:30 a.m.: Listen to favorite music, get dressed and washed. (When I start having any sort of psych problems, personal hygiene is the first thing to go, and it helps me feel sane again to put on clean clothes and brush my hair.)

11 a.m.: Take bus to nature park. I like to go for bus rides when I'm starting to feel crazy, because they're low stress and comforting, there's someone responsible behind the wheel, and it's not as lonely as hanging out at home alone.

12 p.m.: Go for a hike. Hiking is good exercise, uses up excess energy, and feels spiritually meaningful to me. Plus it feels pretty badass to tell people I blew off work/school to climb Mt. Doom.

4 p.m.: Finished hike, have lunch at the coffee shop next to the bus stop. I don't eat out very often, so I really feel cared for and special when I do—and that's the whole point of the mental-health day.

5 p.m.: Write in journal while waiting for the bus. Writing is the way I keep my brain from exploding, and I especially need to make time for it when I'm feeling weird.

6:30 p.m.: Get home after nice long bus ride. Hang out with roommates. Feeling pretty good.

8:30 p.m.: Have a late, healthy dinner.

10 p.m.: Get to bed early for a good sleep before going back to school/work in the morning. Mental-health day successful.

9

VOICES NOT IN YOUR HEAD
DEALING WITH FRIENDS AND FAMILY

Telling someone you have bipolar is like showing them your snake-eating-a-unicorn tattoo for the first time. What if they think you're crazy? What if you're embarrassed? What if it slips out in public? Can I get this thing removed?

Solid friendships and relationships are the foundation of any healthy life, especially a life with bipolar. This chapter covers everything to do with your nearest and dearest.

PART 1: THE DATING GAME

Dating someone when you have bipolar is a lot like dating someone when you don't have bipolar, except when you have bipolar, your significant other (or S.O.) has to be cool with things like meds, depression, and occasionally being locked out of his own house at 1 a.m. while you spontaneously rewallpaper his bedroom. You also need to decide when your S.O.'s making a valid observation ("You seem manic") and when she's just using your diagnosis to score points and win arguments.

A lot of the time, the fact that you have bipolar disorder will be completely unnoticeable to whoever you're dating, but for the times when it does come up, you need an S.O. who's insightful, understanding, and well-informed.

"WHEN AND HOW SHOULD I TELL MY NEW BOY- OR GIRLFRIEND I'M BIPOLAR?"

When should you make out with someone for the first time? On the first date? On your wedding night? Anytime, as long as you've both brushed your teeth?

People can say what they want; rules about when to kiss someone (or tell someone you're bipolar) are meaningless. What really matters is the spirit in which you do it. On night one you can have beautiful, happy tongue hockey or guilty, unhappy tongue hockey, and the difference isn't anything inherent to night one, but the fact that you chose to establish certain feelings around it.

Similarly, when and how you tell your potential love monkey you have bipolar aren't as important as the attitude you communicate when you do it. If you're squeamish and tiptoe around the subject, you'll burden it with unnecessary secrecy and anxiety. If you're upfront and casual about it, you'll establish that it's cool to talk about.

No matter how nervous you feel about telling your S.O. you have bipolar, remember that you're the one choosing to be nervous, and you can just as easily choose *not* to be nervous about it. Trust me: if you establish an attitude of openness and positivity about bipolar in your relationship, you'll be doing yourself a huge favor. Once you've communicated that you're cool with being bipolar, your S.O. will catch on, and he/she/it too will be nonchalant. It will be cool to talk about it, cool to ask you questions, because when something's in the open, it's not so scary anymore. (If they're not cool, then do as Dan Savage says and DTMFA.)

You don't need a special script or special time to bring up bipolar. Rehearsing a mental script implies that you're still kind of anxious about it, so if you're doing that, you should really be working on your own attitude before you bring it up. I know what it's like: it took me two months of taking "heart medication," going "to the post office," and rehearsing mental scripts before telling my first post-diagnosis boyfriend I was bipolar. All that planning and worrying filled the subject of bipolar with extremely awkward mojo. When I finally told him, my terrified expression was more disturbing to him than the news itself. I burned with embarrassment for days afterwards, and we never talked about it again.

Over the next few years, as I became more confident and less of a spazz case (kind of), my approach to bipolar changed—and so, naturally, did the mojo surrounding it. I told my current boyfriend I have bipolar on the night we met. It came up naturally, as part of a fun, casual discussion and has remained a completely comfortable subject ever since. As long as I complete his "mood checklist worksheet" every night and agree to random blood-serum-Seroquel inspections, he doesn't even make me sit in the "quiet box." Not anymore.

Do as Chinese author Wang Xiabo does in his fiction: treat heavy things lightly and light things heavily. Bipolar can be a heavy thing; don't weigh it down further by adding burdens of guilt and anxiety.

"WHY IS IT SO HARD TO TELL SOMEONE I'M BIPOLAR?"

When you disclose a mental illness to someone, you get freaked out because you can't control their reaction or their image of you. You worry that they'll look at you differently, think you're stupid or weird, or that there will be an awkward silence and you'll start babbling to fill it. You take responsibility for the other person's reaction, when it's entirely out of your control. You're like a tennis player on one side of the court, trying to direct the other player's serve through telekinesis.

The truth is, you're worried for good reasons. People *do* react badly to being told somebody they are interested in (and could potentially be "stuck with" for a while) might not always be "the same person." That's a scary thought. So yeah, you might not always get the reaction you want. But the less you stress, the better it'll go.

And guess what? Hormones'll do the talking for you. People are pretty irrational. Even if it were a *terrible* idea to date you, and if they were told that every two months you turned into a bloodthirsty, evil, Satan-worshipping dragon that tore the countryside asunder and listened to tween pop, they'd probably find a way to rationalize liking you: "Well, it's only Satan." "C'mon, it's just the Jonas Brothers." If someone really likes you, they're probably going to find a way to bend this new information into *still* liking you.

Successfully telling someone about your bipolar disorder doesn't mean controlling or anticipating their reaction, but being completely comfortable with not having control. Let's say you tell your boyfriend you have bipolar, and in response he cries, vomits, and tries to roll and smoke his own underwear. So what? Eventually, that particular moment in your life will be over, and the next thing you know you'll all be laughing and getting a burrito. Or you'll decide he's neurotic and controlling and dump his sorry ass. Instead of wasting your life being freaked out and nervous, just be cool. Be cool! And realize, on every level, that if other people aren't cool, that's their problem and their choice. Freedom is nothing more than the constant, thrilling awareness that you're free, that you choose your own attitude from moment to moment—and that you can't control other peoples' choices.

"SCREW THAT, HOW DO I TELL MY BOYFRIEND I HAVE BIPOLAR?"

Sigh. Fine. Rehearse in front of a mirror one of the following:

- (at a lull in any conversation) "Hey, did I ever tell you I have bipolar?"
- (in the middle of passionate sex) "Hey, did I ever tell you I'm bipolar? But, like, I'm only type II, and so its not like, type I which you may have seen in movies and stuff, and …Oh! Oh! Oh!"
- (when you're reading the paper together) "That Zyprexa scandal's some fucked up shit! I have bipolar."

PROS AND CONS OF COHABITATION

I don't believe in doing a lot of sobering, cost-benefit-analysis forethought stuff, which is why I moved in with my boyfriend ten days after I met him. But what I lack in prudence I make up for in luck: not only has living with Seth been a constant source of happiness, but it's also had an unexpected stabilizing effect on my mood cycles. I think the social-rhythm-therapy people are onto something: having a stable rhythm of daily interaction with

Seth, after a lifetime of alternating bursts of isolation and sociability, was the missing link for me. I even sleep better when he falls asleep easily next to me. Not to mention the fact that exercise and regular bedtimes are much easier with the lure of a beloved partner to do them with.

But take heed: I'm pretty sure the move-in gods dispense bliss and havoc in equal measure, and if you're the thinking type, here are some points to consider before shacking up.

Moving in together will definitely affect the following areas: sleep habits, eating habits, habit habits, and social rhythm. Moving in together *will* affect each of these categories to some degree. If you need absolute, nonnegotiable control over any one of them, you should proceed with extreme caution.

SLEEP HABITS: Can she get behind going to sleep at the same time every night? What time can we agree on? Can I deal with agreeing on a bedtime that's earlier or later than I prefer? Do we always need to go to bed together, or are we comfortable going to bed at separate times? Do I take my sleep meds whenever I feel like, or do I let my partner know before taking meds that make me drowsy? Do I need absolute quiet and darkness to sleep, and is this possible if we live together?

Set up your living space so that even if one of you goes to bed early, the other one can still move around and do stuff without disturbing them. A curtain around the bed is good for blocking light, and earplugs and a sleeping mask work wonders. Have an alternate sleeping place, like a couch or spare bed, for nights when one of you is sleeping restlessly or is too hot or cold for the main bed's temperature level. Finally, don't be unnecessarily rigid, but don't sacrifice your health. If you need to get eight hours of sleep in order to stay level, let your partner know how important it is.

EATING HABITS: If your new roomie/paramour is the kind of person who skips breakfast, has a chocolate croissant and a shot of espresso for lunch, and orders an elaborate Indian buffet at 3 a.m., it can be really hard not to do the same. Sticking to your own particular food plan (and budget) is tricky, but important if your sanity depends on regular mealtimes and lots of oatmeal.

If you move in with someone who drinks more than you, you'll probably start drinking more. If you move in with someone who drinks less than you, you'll probably start drinking less. Same applies for stuff like smoking, recreational drugs, exercise, and TV watching. Think about: Do I want this person's habits? Can I hold my own, or will I drift towards their habits? Look, I don't mean to dispense general-purpose relationship advice—just asking you to keep these things in mind.

SOCIAL RHYTHM: Is he going to have a bunch of friends over every night? Do you feel pressure to constantly hang out together, or can you comfortably be around each other while doing separate things? Are you going to have other roommates? Are there separate parts of the house or apartment where you can escape to if you feel like being alone while she's hanging out with people? Do you need a lot of time to yourself, or do you want to be around her all the time?

NOTES: At best, cohabitation can drastically stabilize and improve your life. At worst, it can turn you into a quivering ball of psychotic putty. Make sure you always have a place you can go to be by yourself—be it a room in your house or at your parents' house, a friend's basement, or even a campsite in the woods.

WAYS TO MAKE YOUR BIPOLAR DISORDER EASIER ON YOUR PARTNER

- *Take care of yourself.*

  There's nothing more frustrating than watching someone who *could* be healthy and happy dig themselves into a hole. Your partner will feel much better if he/she can tell you're taking care of yourself. So take your meds and lay off the 3 a.m. whiskey binges, already.

- *Tell them when you think you're cycling.*

  They may have already noticed—or not. If they have, they'll be relieved to know that *you know* that you're cycling, and are taking steps to maintain insight. If they hadn't noticed, it can help to know they hadn't, because it tells you that you aren't way off track yet.

- *Keep other support networks current.*

  Don't stop hanging out with your friends now that you have a significant other. Keep going to your support group, your yoga class, and Sunday dinner at your aunt's house so you don't depend on your S.O. exclusively for love and support. That way when you're manic, you'll have more than one person to tell about your plan for infiltrating the White House.

- *Keep them informed.*

  Be open and forthcoming about how you're doing. Keep them in the loop about which meds you're taking and their side effects. There's no need to start a constant RSS feed about your mood states, but checking in when something comes up is reasonable. It's way less stressful to be with someone who's upfront about being depressed or manic than someone who tries to hide all their feelings.

- *Be gentle.*

  Both depression and (hypo)mania can make you irritable and prone to lashing out at your partner. Take special care to be gentle with their feelings when you're depressed or (hypo)manic. And remember that they need back rubs just as much as you do.

PART 2: FRIENDS AND FAMILY

Your friends and family are the people you eat with, gossip with, watch *Star Wars* marathons with, and generally like. They're also your most important support network. Your relationship with them goes two ways: they support you, but they also need your support. In this respect, they're not like psychiatrists. If you don't love them back, your relationship will wither. They have a vested interest in your being sane, healthy, and happy—you're more fun that way than when you're unstable and crazy. Take care of your friendships, and you'll have a much better time of life. Help your friends and family understand what bipolar is, and you'll all be able to take better care of each other.

FRIENDS AND FAMILY: KEEPING THEM INFORMED AND HAPPY

"WAS I THE LAST PERSON TO REALIZE I WAS CRAZY? DID ALL MY FRIENDS AND FAMILY KNOW IT ALL ALONG?": Most people don't recognize the signs of mental illness. Unless you're out on the street in your boxers, muttering to yourself about aliens (and even then, some people will just think you're fun to have around at, you know, space parties and stuff), most people won't connect things like mood swings and insomnia to mental illness until you get diagnosed. And then all the little oddities they couldn't quite put their finger on "suddenly make sense." My friend started med school this year, and halfway through the first semester his roommate, who had no history of mental illness, was hospitalized for psychosis. He was shocked; he'd never seen anyone "go crazy" before and couldn't believe he'd cheerfully, cluelessly witnessed his roommate's psychosis without catching on that something was wrong or reaching out to help. Similarly, when I had my first struggles with bipolar, none of my friends recognized the signs. But when I told them the diagnosis, they said that, in hindsight, it explained a lot of things.

In the wake of a bipolar diagnosis, parents, friends, and relatives who didn't recognize the signs of mental illness are probably thinking:

> "I thought he was just stressed out by exams."
>
> "I tried to be nice to her when I saw her."
>
> "I just thought he was drunk."
>
> "I thought she really was pregnant with Steven Colbert's baby."
>
> "He did always talk about a lot of weird stuff."
>
> "I thought she was just working too hard."
>
> "He seemed perfectly normal."
>
> "She was always so cheerful. I can't believe she was depressed."
>
> "If only I'd paid more attention, I could have gotten him help sooner."
>
> "I had absolutely no idea."

Your friends and family might know less about bipolar than you think, so explain it to them. Lend them a book about bipolar. (How about this one? On second thought, don't lend. *Buy* them books. Buy *all* of them books. How about this one?) Most people who don't have one are fascinated by mental illness. They've never experienced mania or psychosis and would love to hear your stories. (Without warning, feed them high doses of magic mushrooms. Ha! Now they understand; serves them right.) Close friends often feel privileged to be offered a window into this very raw, private part of your existence. And once they understand that your depression isn't moodiness and your hypomania isn't belligerence, they won't be as hurt or confused when these happen.

You can also take a parent, friend, or significant other with you into the doctor or psychiatrist's office, so they can ask questions and feel more involved in your treatment. If you ever get hospitalized, it will be good to have a friend or parent around who knows your doctor and can help make good decisions—decisions you might be too crazy to make on your own.

Being open and well-informed about bipolar yourself will make it much easier for your friends and family to be open and well-informed too. If they have preconceptions of or biases against mental illness, talking about it will help them realize where and how they're wrong. You can't force people to understand, but you can leave the door open.

DEALING WITH PARENTS

Your parents' reaction to finding out you have bipolar can be more intense and harder to deal with than anyone else's. Parents get all sorts of stressed when they find out their kid has a mental illness. Guilt, anger, worry, disappointment, and overprotectiveness are just the beginning. And why not? After all, they just failed as parents, right?

Some parents are awesome; they understand, help when appropriate, back off when appropriate, stay cool. And some parents flip their lids and suddenly look at you like you've replaced their perfect child with a demonic imposter. Instead of being mad or hurt at their reactions, try to understand where they're coming from. Maybe they need support only you can give. Maybe you need cash only they can give. It works out. Here's what they might be feeling:

- *Guilt*

  Some parents feel guilty for passing on the bipolar gene to their kids. Maybe your mom's mom was bipolar. So Mom has seen how it can mess you up, and she feels terrible for putting you at risk for it. Guilt can often masquerade as anger or resentment.

- *Anger*

  Parents who don't understand that bipolar is genetic and out of your control might respond with anger:" How can you do this to us? You're such a screw-up!" They mistakenly assume that you're "doing it on purpose" or "making a scene," and might demand that you stop doing that bipolar thing the same way you tell someone to stop leaving dishes on the counter or knock off that racket in the garage. As Yoda tells us, anger is a close cousin to fear: bipolar disorder is an animal they don't recognize, they don't know what the frack they're supposed to do when they run into one, and the only surefire plan is to pick up a big stick and threaten it.

- *Worry*

  "Do you want to move back home? Should we send your big brother out there to take care of you?" Parents worry—especially if you live far away, and they can't see you to know you're OK. They worry that you're more crazy than you really are, that you can't take care of yourself, and that you'll crack without a constant supply of homemade cookies. (That last one might be true.)

- *A need to take control*

  There's nothing more annoying than being asked if you've taken your meds when you always take your meds, or being asked about your mood every day like a toddler being asked by the nanny if he's made a poo. (Side note: it's even *more* annoying being asked if you've taken your meds when you *haven't* been taking your meds. But maybe they have a point—maybe you should come down from that tree and take your meds.) Many parents turn to over-controllingness to deal with their own feelings of fear and worry in the face of your apparently "out of control" disorder.

- *Disappointment or anxiety*

  "What will this mean for medical school?" "Can you still take over the business?" "You were in hospital through the entire football season!" "Well, call me again next semester, I guess." Parents hang a lot of hopes on their kids, and your bipolar disorder is one of those things that makes them realize your life is yours, not theirs. Just as you have to face a future of bipolar episodes, they're faced with a new set of worries about the future—some justified, some not.

Other possible aspects of parental flip-out:

- *False beliefs about bipolar*

  The summer after I was diagnosed, I was working in Jasper, Alberta, and looking into buying my first beater car so I could get around to hiking trailheads. I found out from a nearby relative that my parents had alerted them to the perils of my condition: "Don't let Hilary drive. She's got monomania!" I was highly insulted—'m a very prudent driver—and was outraged that my parents were "warning" relatives about me (I later realized that the original words were probably nothing like the message my aunt seemed to remember these things get bungled all the time). When people don't know much about a subject that's suddenly relevant to them, they sometimes start to pull beliefs out of thin air, or cobble together things they've heard, things they've read, and things they made up from scratch. Often this is out of a spirit of protectiveness. Let them down gently. ("Seriously, Dad, I only drive 200 mph at 3 a.m. when there's like nobody else on the road.")

- *Non-responsiveness*

  You've reached out to them, and all you get is radio static. If you bring up your bipolar disorder, one of your parents changes the subject abruptly. "Don't they understand what a big deal this is?" you wonder.

  Non-responsiveness is probably the most confusing reaction you can get from a parent, because it gives you nothing to chew on, lean on, or even fight against. Some parents just have a hard time talking about sensitive things, —or they're afraid you'll get mad if they ask you questions. The best thing you can do in this situation is to keep on being open and communicative, and not get frustrated by their perceived lack of response. Maintaining this stance is not easy, but at least it's not destructive. Some parents eventually come around and open up about it, and with others the subject of mental illness remains a closed book. In the latter case, it's especially important to find a friend or counselor with whom you can spill your guts about your moods and meds.

In order to deal with all of these reactions effectively, most parents need three things: involvement, information, and reassurance. If your parents want to feel involved in your treatment, let them go right ahead and spend hours on the phone with the health insurance company. Most moms and dads would be thrilled if their kids asked them for advice, so even if you don't take it, make your dad feel good and ask him what he does when he's depressed. If you're parents are totally ignorant about what bipolar is, nurture them with information. If they worry about you constantly, throw them a bone; invite them over for dinner so they can see how happy you are, how well you're doing, and how bad a cook you are.

No matter how hysterical or inappropriate your parents' reaction is, don't let it get to you. You can only do your best to help them through your diagnosis. The rest is up to them.

DEALING WITH FRIENDS

Friends have slightly different needs than parents. They don't need to know if their offspring will still make it to medical school and don't want to know the names of every doctor you've seen. Your friends need a fun, cool person to hang out with—a person who cares about them as much as they care about you. How can you keep your friendships balanced when you frequently have manic or depressive episodes that need a lot of attention, and they just don't?

Most of the things I wrote about parents and significant others also apply to friends. Establish an attitude of openness about bipolar. Keep them informed and involved in your life. If they get mad at you for being manic, or feel hurt when you get depressed, understand that it's because they don't know much about mental illness. Help them learn. A friend who doesn't know anything about bipolar might think you're drunk when you're really manic, or that you're mad at them when you don't return their phone calls when you're depressed. It's easy to misinterpret these things. Be gentle with your friends' feelings, and forgive them if they misunderstand.

You're going to need to work out how much of your mood cycles to share with your friends. Do your friends need a play-by-play recap of your every depression, your every hypomanic discovery? You want to let your friends into your life, but you also don't want to be the hypochondriac uncle who calls up the whole family every time he has indigestion. It's best to find a happy medium. If your bipolar is acting up, mention it, but don't let it dominate your relationship.

LAST THOUGHTS ON FRIENDS, PARENTS, AND SIGNIFICANT OTHERS

Getting diagnosed with bipolar is a great opportunity to become a more open person, a more honest person, a more caring person. Having all these people care about you makes you realize how much you value them—and how much you can return their love. If you can be open about bipolar, you can be open about other touchy things—(dirty family secrets, anyone?). Being "crazy" is a great excuse to speak your mind and ask awkward questions—it can even be a catalyst for taking big steps like coming out of the closet. You can use bipolar as an excuse for cracking open taboo issues in your life, and if doing so completely backfires, just blame it on the mania!

10

HIPPIE SHIT THAT ACTUALLY WORKS
HERBS, WILDERNESS TIME, AND OTHER WAYS TO HELP YOU KEEP YOUR SHIT TOGETHER

As you go through life, you'll find yourself doing three kinds of things to deal with your bipolar symptoms: the things you do because your doctor says so (like taking your pills), the things you do because your mom says so (like taking your bath), and the things you do because they feel just right. We're here to talk about this third category: the whimsical, spiritual, completely unscientific little habits and rituals you do throughout the day or year to deal with depression, make sense of mania, and basically keep your head together. We're here to light some incense, put on some trance music, and dance with our spirit animals. We're here to play bongo drums with some long-haired dudes we met on the beach. Welcome to the chapter on hippie shit. Now let's self-actualize, man.

MEDITATION AND DETACHMENT

Guru says, "All we have are random, impersonal circumstances and the booby prize called free will!"

Buddhism teaches you even if you're in a straitjacket, you can still be free as a bird if you practice detachment. Detachment is the ultimate expression of not giving a shit—not giving a shit if you're scared, not giving a shit if you're comfortable or not, not giving a shit if you're rich or poor, or happy or sad, or even in excruciating pain. The Buddhist response to mania and depression is to smile peacefully and say, "Oh, depression is happening. So what? Mania is happening. So what? I'm in a straitjacket. Oh well, this rather humorous situation, like all situations, will eventually pass."

When you meditate, you observe your thoughts and physical sensations without reacting to them. At first, you notice yourself becoming grouchy if your back hurts. You realize that you've handed this puny little backache the power to make you feel bad. What a bitch! The next time your back hurts, you simply observe it without becoming grouchy. As you practice this nonreactive observation again and again, you gradually free yourself. You become happier, because you've stopped handing other things, people, and situations the power to make you sad. If you go far enough with meditation, someone could stab you in the face, and you'd be no more upset than if they'd just handed you a birthday cake.

Here are examples of detachment in everyday life:

Situation	Attached reaction	Detached reaction
A bear is chasing you.	Fear, panic, pants wetting	Calm, happiness
You're getting rained on.	Irritation, discomfort	Calm, happiness
You're starving.	Craving, crankiness	Calm, happiness

Meditation is also useful for calming your mind, dealing with anxiety, and learning to sit still for longer than fifteen seconds at a time.

FUN WITH HERBS

Some people find it fun or interesting to supplement their pharmaceutical medications with herbal remedies concocted by ancient tribes of dirty hippies and sold today at your local alternative health store. Herbs work subtly. They're not tranquilizers. Don't drink a cup of chamomile tea and expect the same effects as Klonopin. Chamomile is not Klonopin. Marijuana might be Klonopin. Klonopin might be Klonopin. But chamomile tea is chamomile tea. Appreciate herbal remedies for what they are: mild, gentle. If their effects are more of the placebo variety, that's cool. Evidence of the effectiveness of all of the following herbs is *mondo inconclusivo,* so mainly consider them a tool for tricking yourself into feeling calmer or sleepier or whatever.

Valerian might be the world's oldest insomnia remedy: the first recorded use of valerian for insomnia was in the second century. Nowadays you can find it in tea, extract, or pill form, often combined with other herbs with soothing properties, like lavender. I once found a valerian-lavender concoction you were supposed to apply to the soles of your feet. Now that's some hippie shit.

Kava kava is a beverage made of dried kava root and drunk ceremonially in Pacific islands like Samoa and Hawai'i. It's the only one of the herbs here discussed that has actually been shown in research to have a more significant effect than a placebo—namely, mild sedation and better sleep. You can get it in powder form at Pacific Island grocery stores. It doesn't exactly taste good, but it makes your lips feel numb, which is kind of cool.

Common skullcap is thought to be a mild sedative. And guess what? You can smoke it! Sweet, man!

Damiana is also thought to have sedative properties. And dig this—you can smoke it too!

St. John's wort is pretty well hyped for depression by now. You can buy commercial preparations of it in most grocery stores. It doesn't interact well with MAOI inhibitors, so don't mix your meds. And you can't smoke it. I've read that, like other antidepressants, it can induce mania or hypomania in people who have a predisposition towards those states. So definitely consult with your doctor before worting it up.

Marijuana for, um, medicinal purposes, is now legal in thirteen states. For many people with bipolar disorder, smoking a joint really is "good medicine": it can lighten depression, help you sleep, improve your appetite, and calm you down if you're edgy and hypomanic. Plus, weed has the bonus of being the one "med" that makes reggae music sound better (when's the last time lithium did that?). Like any other medicine, marijuana has different effects on different people: some people find that using it makes them more depressed, or aggravates their insomnia. And while there has been no proven link between bong-hits and bipolar, some doctors think that smoking weed makes it harder to deal with symptoms (other doctors think it's great!).

WILDERNESS TIME

I've heard that when put in survival situations, even suicidal people will fight for their lives. Some prisons dump their inmates into isolated wilderness for rehabilitation; summer camps for troubled kids and teens are also fond of this technique. Why is solitude in the wilderness so effective at sparking deep insights and life reckonings? My bet's on the fact that it pares you down to the abilities you have in your own body and your own mind. You don't have other people around to help you out or piss you off. You don't have machines or tools. You realize the extent to which your life is in your own hands —or out of them, if the weather is anything to go by.

If you have no purpose in life, going into the wilderness gives you an instant purpose: survival. Your only job, from day to day, is to take care of your basic needs for food, water, shelter, and heat, and your only company is yourself. You have plenty of time and opportunity to observe the changing nature of nature itself. You witness a sunrise and sunset every morning and evening. You see clouds forming, dropping rain, and breaking into blue sky. Your body feels keenly how the day starts out cool, warms up gradually, and cools down again as it turns to evening—something you might never feel if you spend all your time in a climate-controlled environment. If you're near the ocean, you witness the tide going in and out each day. The moon changes a little bit each night. And the plants and animals around you change visibly too. Even over the course of a single week, you can watch a seedling sprout out of its pod, a flower bloom, berries ripen, the progression of a bird's nest or beaver's dam being built.

With all this change going on around you, the wheels of your mind slow down and stop pushing forward an endless stream of concerns and mental chatter, and you're eventually forced to surrender to the fact that the world keeps on going no matter what you do.

Some people think that cities contribute to mental illness, because they're environments of intense, non-stop stimulation that can also be completely impersonal. The theory goes that the structure of a city—the primacy of motor vehicles over people, the deluge of words and images, and the endless passage of people with whom we never make eye contact or acknowledge in any way—is pathological. There's a collective fantasy of fame and urgency: you have to be someone, and you have to eat, drink, buy, or do something stimulating at all times. You start to feel like what you do with your life is really important, when at the same time, nobody in the endless stream of strangers knows you or cares. You feel pressure to go to a show, to meet people, to entertain yourself, to be happy. Who's standing over your shoulder keeping tabs on how entertained and happy you are? This is the collective delusion of a city: that someone gives a hoot about all the rad, awesome parties you go to.

When I get depressed, I weep and feel intensely guilty for not being famous. I feel, *insanely*, that my not being famous is letting down a slew of imaginary onlookers who are very, very disappointed at my lack of progress. Fame—not marriage, money, or happiness—is the ultimate endgame. On the other side of the coin, when I'm hypomanic I feel very optimistic that my (trivial) day-to-day activities and projects have a famous flavor to them.

Going into the wilderness dissolves this illusory fame game and reveals it for what it is: completely arbitrary. A lightning storm doesn't care how many hits a day your website gets. A prowling grizzly bear doesn't care how many people recognize you at the bar. Nature's failure to recognize you and tailor itself to your greatness breaks down your narcissism pretty fast. You realize the imaginary tally you carry around in your head has no inherent value and is completely disposable, pure ether. It's disconcerting, but ultimately the most comforting balm I know is the knowledge that I am no one. Just another green shoot rising and getting eaten by a deer. The universe swirls on.

ECSTATIC DANCING

I recently read a book by Gabrielle Roth called *Maps to Ecstasy* and have become temporarily obsessed. The book talks about movement and rhythm as the core of life. Roth suggests there are five basic rhythms to life and that we need to acknowledge and dance all our rhythms in order to be fully realized people. Sounds kinda like a metaphor for bipolar, doesn't it? Roth's idea is that instead of suppressing or denying any of our rhythms, we should literally dance them—dance flowingly, dance chaotically, dance our anger and sadness as well as our joy. Try it: next time you're getting (hypo)manic or depressed, put on some music and express your experience with dance. Especially try it if you're getting depressed. I don't know about you, but I already dance a lot when I'm getting speedy, and the fact that depression doesn't normally lend itself to dance makes the dance even *more* potent.

GOOD WORDS

Poets have high emotional quotients. I trust the motherfuckers. When it comes to wild emotions, God knows they've been there and undoubtedly further. The fruits of their experience, the poems, remind me that you can come out of any situation with wisdom and grace, with flair and humor. When I get hypomanic or depressed, I go to my own personal oracle: poems by Rumi and Rainer Maria Rilke, and passages from an Annie Dillard book. They're short, potent reminders of the kind of attitude I aspire to have towards life; they're words of strength and playfulness, insight and wisdom. They remind me of the many alternate ways I can choose to confront a certain emotion or situation, before I lose my head and sink too far into a certain mental state.

Having emergency poems or quotes to read when you're getting depressed or manic is great, because they remind you of all the wisdom you tend to throw out the window when the wolf is at the door. When people get into trouble, the first thing that often happens is they forget all the careful planning and in-case-of-emergency steps they decided to take in the event of a disaster. So at a time when you're not actively depressed or (hypo)manic, choose some verses, passages, or quotes from a text that resonates with you and that will help you through when you're having an episode. Copy them down and keep them posted somewhere where you won't forget to read them. Good words are good medicine.

GOOD MUSIC

Music is *powerful*. It can make your brain light up and twinkle when you thought you would never smile again, or it can soothe you to sleep when you're too agitated to close your eyes. Plus, the music you listen to will inevitably affect your mental narrative. Years later, you'll stumble across the music you listened to when you were first diagnosed with bipolar disorder, and, just like when you hear the song they played at your junior prom, you'll find yourself swimming in nostalgia. (Whenever I hear Modest Mouse, I get flashbacks of rainy all-night bike rides and can practically smell the old house I used to live in.)

Listening to the right music for your mood is like talking to a friend who really, really understands you— which, during a depressed or hypo/manic episode, is just what you need. Keep two emergency playlists of songs and tunes that trigger powerful emotions in you—one list for depression, one for (hypo)mania. When you need something to help you through, just turn up the volume.

Some ideas follow.

DEPRESSION PLAYLIST

- gangsta rap to remind you how tough and badass you are
- sad songs that help you feel your emotions without making you wanna kill yourself
- Tibetan chanting—calming and soothing, and you don't need to understand the words
- companionable songs that feel like old friends, like "Pack Up Your Sorrows" by Mimi and Richard Farina, to keep you company if you feel lonely.
- electro music with a steady beat that helps your mind dissolve. (Electro music also makes great walking music.)

HYPOMANIA/MANIA PLAYLIST

- ragas
- music with binaural beats to slow your mind down and help you sleep
- slow music to help keep you from speeding while you're driving
- happy songs that help you enjoy your high
- fugues by J. S. Bach: your increased focus will help you hear all sorts of connections and patterns you never heard before.
- the *Goldberg Variations* by J. S. Bach: they were written as a cure for a king's insomnia and are intended to be calming.

ANIMAL THERAPY

Full disclosure: I never had pets growing up, and whenever I heard people talking about how their beloved Ralph or Skooter helped them get through the day, I secretly thought it was crap. But a few months ago I took home a pair of abandoned kittens I found in the park, and having finally experienced what it's like to live with warm, fuzzy animals, I've changed my Scrooge-like opinions. Animals are great, especially if you're prone to the highs and lows of a mood disorder. Having a friendly creature around helps dispel loneliness, provides structure and responsibility, and gives you a guaranteed playmate or exercise buddy. Some people with bipolar disorder even have service dogs (protected by the Americans with Disabilities Act!) who bark when it's time for meds and nuzzle them when they're having a panic attack. If you can't own a pet, try volunteering at an animal shelter or making friends with a neighbor's dog, cat, horse, pig, or llama. The love they give is definitely worth the slobber and hairballs.

MASSAGE

Sometimes, we manic-depressos get so overwhelmed by the mental anguish of depression that we forget to seek relief for our physical selves. But our bodies need relief just as much as our minds. Depression can make your head ache, your muscles tense, or your body feel completely senseless. A good massage can help you come back to life, at least temporarily. Ask your friend or lover to give you a hand, foot, shoulder, or head massage (you might have to offer a trade!) Then relax and focus on the positive physical sensations. Sometimes when I'm depressed, even paying extra attention while I brush my hair or take a shower is enough to relieve some of the mental anguish and remind myself I have a body.

Psychedelics exist. Plenty of people take them. There's no point pretending that people with mental illnesses don't take them. Yet it's practically impossible to find good information about psychedelics and bipolar disorder because everyone who writes a book or puts up a website has to decorate their information with more disclaimers than a Christmas tree has twinkle lights, just to cover their backs. You find the kind of ambiguous statement like, "I'm bipolar and shrooms work great for me and heal my depression. But you should never, ever drop shrooms if you're bipolar because they can trigger shit in your brain that will screw you up permanently." Well, will they or won't they? Is taking psychedelics riskier for people with bipolar, because our brain chemistry is easily triggered into episodes, or are people with bipolar better equipped to take psychedelics than the general population, because we're already experienced navigators of alternate realities? So-called studies on the subject are no better than subjective accounts. Everyone's hands are tied.

The only conclusions I can draw after hours of research are that psychedelics might have a bad interaction with your meds, and they may or may not trigger a psychotic, depressive, or manic episode. Real helpful, right?

Experienced trippers say the most important thing about taking psychedelics is being stable, able to keep your cool, and in the right setting—*not* whether or not you have a diagnosis. The most important thing about being able to drive a fire truck is being calm, alert, and well trained in fire-truck driving—qualities a person with bipolar can possess as easily as a person without. When making the decision to drop or not to drop, evaluate yourself thoroughly and honestly: What are your abilities, your state of mind, your personal history and current level of stability? Is this a good time to risk triggering an episode? Have you taken this kind of mushroom/cactus/button before? Do your best to research whether or not there's a danger of nasty interactions with whatever meds you're on. And if in doubt, don't do it. Doubt and apprehension guarantee a bad trip.

I'm not experienced enough with psychedelics to give any more advice on the subject or wax poetic about how the fractal kingdom expanded my mind beyond the limits of reality. I know people with bipolar disorder who dose regularly and seem completely fine and unaffected, and people with bipolar disorder whose psychedelic use temporarily made their lives a living hell. There doesn't seem to be a single rule.

P.S. Excessive rumination about whether a drug will "screw you up for life" can give the experience more import and drama than it really deserves. Every day, all kinds of people take shrooms and acid and peyote and whatnot. Normal people, mundane people, just boring ol' people. Fifteen-year-old high schoolers and thirty-year-old ski instructors. Your history prof. All around the world, people who have taken psychedelic drugs are turning out OK, turning out to be losers, turning out to be successful, turning out to be psychotic—the whole range. What's the big deal? You're just another grain of sand on a vast beach. Sooner or later even the most impactful psychedelic experience fades into kitsch. So chill out.

11

HELL IS FINDING GOOD INSURANCE
HOW TO GET YOUR ASS COVERED
IN TROUBLED TIMES

If you live in Canada or Germany or some other sane country with universal health care, you can rip this chapter out of the book, tear it into shreds, and dance around in the confetti, because you don't need to worry about buying private health insurance. If you live in the United States, read on with trepidation.

Just so you know, health insurance companies hate you.

Now that that little unpleasantry is over with, let's talk about health insurance. Health insurance is something you need, if not because you have bipolar then because you have as good a chance as anybody of breaking your leg or coming down with mono. Unfortunately, having a bipolar diagnosis makes it damn near impossible to get individual health insurance in some states. Even though you might be a perfectly prudent, mild person, insurers see you as a high risk. Aren't people with bipolar disorder always running their cars off cliffs and mainlining heroin in the grocery-store lineup? Insurers want to cover people who don't need insurance, and they're afraid that if they cover you, you'll skip off to a mental hospital and cost them thousands of dollars.

That's not to say that it's completely impossible to get insured. There are ways to get insured—some of them expensive, some of them sneaky, some of them obvious—and if you proceed patiently and don't get too flustered if the first few tries fail, you can eventually reach a state of happy insurement.

This chapter will give you a few tools to help you wade through the swamp of finding health care if you aren't covered by your school or employer. I can't give you advice on specific plans or providers because they all vary by state. But at the end of this chapter you should feel empowered to take a stab at getting your health insurance situation figured out. As some of you might be aware, President Barack Obama has promised to establish universal health care in America during his first term. In addition to advice on navigating the current health-care system, we'll have a look at some of the proposed health-care reforms and what they'll mean for people with mental illnesses.

PART ONE: TALKING THE TALK

Before you start reading a bunch of health insurance policies, you need to be familiar with a few basic terms. If you don't understand what these terms mean, you won't be able to understand what each plan covers or even how much it's going to cost. Before we go any further, bone up on the following.

PPO

PPO stands for "preferred provider organization." It refers to a bunch of doctors, psychiatrists, dentists, and other medical providers who have made an agreement with your insurance company to provide their services at reduced rates for that company's clients (i.e., you). If you're on a PPO plan, you can find a list of the doctors in your network by going to your health insurance provider's website and typing in your zip code.

HMO

HMO stands for "health maintenance organization." Like *PPO,* it refers to a group of doctors and hospitals that have agreed with an insurance company to serve that company's clients, but unlike a PPO you have to choose one doctor as your primary care physician, and she has to make a referral before you can see a specialist (like a psychiatrist). HMOs are more restrictive than PPOs, but sometimes less expensive.

DEDUCTIBLE

The deductible is the amount of money you have to pay for medical expenses before the insurance company will lift a finger to bail you out. If your deductible is $1,000 (which is quite low), it means you have to pay the first $1,000 of your medical expenses, and the insurance company will pay for whatever expenses you incur beyond that. So if you get hit by a car and the hospital bill is $20,000, the insurer will pay $19,000, and you only need to pay the first $1,000.

Plans with low deductibles are usually more expensive than plans with high deductibles because it's going to cost the insurance company more if you need medical attention. If your deductible is really high, it won't pay for anything except the gravest disasters, but it will be cheaper month to month.

COPAYMENT/COPAY

The copay is the amount you have to pay from your own pocket for a certain service at the time you receive it. For example, if an insurance policy states that a doctor visit has a copayment of $30, it means you have to pay $30 cash money every time you go to the doctor.

Sometimes a plan will say something like "$30 copay before deductible." This means you have to pay $30 each time you see the doctor until you've reached your deductible, at which point you no longer have to pay the $30. For example, if your deductible is $1,000, you would have to go to the doctor thirty-four times (at thirty bucks a pop) before the insurance company would waive the copayment.

A $30 copayment to see a doctor isn't too bad in the great scheme of things. But a copayment can also be a percentage of the total cost for a certain service— for example, a 50 percent copayment on emergency services. This means if you wind up in the emergency room and the bill comes to $5,000, your insurance only pays for $2,500. That's not so bad if you have a low deductible, but bad news if your deductible is high.

OUT-OF-POCKET MAXIMUM

The out-of-pocket maximum is a dollar figure for how much you'd ever have to pay for medical expenses in a year under a particular plan, not including your monthly insurance payments. Most of the time this figure includes the deductible—it might be the same amount as the deductible—but sometimes the insurance company sneaks in an extra amount you'd have to pay on top of the deductible.

GENERICS VERSUS BRAND-NAME DRUGS

Not all plans cover prescription drugs—and if you have bipolar, you're probably taking a handful of those every day. It can be an expensive handful if it's not covered by your insurance. Some plans only cover generic versions of drugs, which is fine for many people, but not so hot if there's no generic version of the drug you want or if you're allergic to an inactive ingredient in the generic version. Before you sign up for any plan, make sure it covers your meds or a generic version thereof at a reasonable rate.

GUARANTEED COVERAGE INSURANCE

Certain states require insurance companies to offer one guaranteed-coverage plan that's available to everyone, regardless of preexisting conditions.

Don't get excited: guaranteed coverage plans are insanely expensive. You don't get a break for having bipolar—far from it. Insurance companies ramp up their rates to cover the "increased risk" of covering reckless ol' you. A standard rate is $350 a month, hardly a "guarantee" of coverage if you can't afford it.

HEALTH SAVINGS ACCOUNT

Many high-deductible individual health insurance plans involve contributing funds to a Health Savings Account

(HSA). An HSA is a tax-free savings account into which you deposit funds earmarked for health care. You can use the money in your HSA to pay your health insurance deductible and other qualified medical expenses like vision and dental. If you use the money in your HSA for other purposes (or for nonqualified medical expenses), you lose the tax advantage and have to pay a 10% tax penalty.

To qualify for an HSA, you must either be enrolled in a high-deductible health insurance plan or have no health insurance coverage whatsoever. If you're enrolled in Medicare or are on somebody else's plan as a dependant, you don't qualify for an HSA.

PART TWO: WALKING THE WALK

Now that you know the lingo, let's walk through the steps of applying for individual health insurance. Company-provided health insurance is covered later in the chapter.

STEP 1: SCOPE OUT YOUR STATE

Every state has different laws regulating private health insurance plans, so your first step is to scope out your own state's health insurance quirks. The Georgetown University Health Policy Institute offers a free, comprehensive guide to health insurance for each state, and their website (*www.healthinsuranceinfo.net*) is absolutely the best resource I've found for getting started. It's important to research your state's laws so you know your rights and are aware of whether or not individual health insurance providers are legally allowed to deny you for preexisting conditions.

STEP 2: RESEARCH PLANS

Go online and browse the policies of health insurance providers in your state. Some websites allow you to compare plans from multiple different providers side-by-side. Check what the monthly rates are, what the deductible and copayments are, and which services are covered by each plan. Some plans exclude mental-health services completely, or cover only a handful of visits to a psychiatrist. Write down a short list of three to five policies that meet your needs and budget.

If you have any questions about what's covered by a certain plan, call the insurance provider to fill in any gaps in your understanding. If you know other people with bipolar disorder, call them up and ask them what their insurance deal is. Do an online search for free clinics in your area, so you know what resources are available to supplement what your insurance doesn't cover.

STEP 3: APPLY

Most insurers have online applications now. When you fill out your application, tell the truth about your medical history and current medication. They're going to review your medical record, and if they find out you lied on your application, they're not legally required to cover you, even if you've been paying the premiums. Health insurance applications can be a pain in the ass to fill out, because they ask a hundred questions about how much alcohol you drink and which diseases you've had and which doctor you've been seeing for checkups. Put on some good music and plow through it.

STEP 4: WAIT

It can take a few weeks for a health insurance companies to process your application. In some cases, you'll get a positive or negative response right away. In other cases, you'll get a letter from the company's underwriters asking for more information about specific details of your medical history. An insurance company might ask for a letter from your psychiatrist, hospital records, or other documents to help them determine how serious your condition is and how stable you are currently. Yes, tracking down all these records is a huge pain in the ass. But your psychiatrist's office has a medical records person (hopefully a friendly one) who can find your records and send copies of relevant documents to the health insurance company. Put on your nicest phone voice, call up your psychiatrist's office, and tell them what you need (it helps to make a list first, so you don't need to call more than once).

Once the health insurance company has snooped around your medical history, you should get a letter in the mail within a couple weeks either accepting or declining your application.

STEP 5: REJOICE OR REBEL

If you get approved for the insurance you want, huzzah! If you get a pile of rejection letters (as you're likely to if you have a bipolar diagnosis), don't panic. You can still get insurance. It's just going to take a little more work, stealth, patience, and persistence.

You, my uninsured friend, need to enter the dog-eat-dog world of . . .

PART 3: HEALTH INSURANCE HACKS

Let's say you've applied for and been rejected from all the normal plans you were considering. You still have a handful of options. By hook or by crook, you can and should get your ass insured, or you can end up deeply in debt if something happens to you. Use one of the following health insurance hacks to get you through the door.

SHORT-TERM HEALTH INSURANCE

Sometimes, health insurance providers don't ask the same questions for short-term insurance as they do for long-term insurance. So even if you don't qualify for reasonably priced long-term insurance, you can sometimes sneak through the cracks and get insurance in six-month chunks—simply because some short-term providers don't bother to ask about mental-health issues. Short-term health insurance is really only useful for disasters like getting hit by a truck. It's often non-renewable, so you'd better hope you don't develop any more chronic conditions once you're on it because it does not cover long-term care. Short-term insurance is good if you're stable enough to not need scheduled doctor visits, if you're in good physical health, and if you really, truly only need insurance for huge emergencies. If you get through the six months without using any services, some providers will let you renew your short-term insurance for another six months. You can bounce around from short-term policy to short-term policy for years before you run out of providers. It's a cheap, legal hack. Cheap because they charge you the same as everybody else ($50 to $100 a month) and legal because if they don't ask, you don't gotta tell. You're covered in the event of a disaster. And if you get the flu, you can go to a free clinic because doctor visits are often not covered by this sort of plan. Don't get a short-term plan if you need to get any mental-health services out of it, because *you won't*. If you need a psychiatrist, you'll need to see her on your dime. So only get short-term health insurance if you're hella stable and physically healthy.

SKOOL

Many colleges offer health plans to their students. Even if you're not a full-time student, you can sometimes get on the college health plan if you're taking as little as one course—even an online course that doesn't require your presence on campus. See what I'm getting at? When you do the math, paying $400 for a college class makes a lot of sense if it gets you cheaper, better insurance that more than pays for itself within a few months. Plus, you get to learn something. Different colleges have different rules about who's eligible for their health plans, so read the fine print before enrolling in Physics 101.

JORB

Tons of employers give health benefits to full-time employees. So you could always, you know, get a full-time job at a company that provides health insurance. Of course, taking care of yourself when you have bipolar disorder can be a full-time job in itself, so if you currently spend the hours between nine and five trying to keep your brain from coming unscrewed, this one may not be an option right now (trust me—*Monster.com* can wait until you're feeling better). It's also not an option if you're a dirty hippie who doesn't want to be a slave for the man. But let's say you find a job you like, and it has the added bonus of covering your ass in terms of health insurance. It could work. Plus, even if you quit the job after a year, you can keep on getting the same health insurance under a federal program called COBRA. It will be more expensive, because your employer won't be subsidizing the premiums, but at least they can't reject you.

'RENTS

In some states, you can stay on your parents' health insurance policy until you're twenty-five years old. Ask your parents if you're eligible to be on their health insurance policy. If so, jump in.

You might also be able to enroll in your parents' plan as a "disabled adult dependant" (not the most flattering term, I know). Eligibility requirements vary, and it's gonna take some phone calls and paperwork, but it's a good option if you qualify.

SELF-EMPLOYMENT

Some states offer group health insurance to "groups of one" (i.e., a single person running his/her own business). These plans are guaranteed coverage, which means they can't deny you based on your medical history. To qualify for a group-of-one medical policy, you have to prove that you've been "in business" for at least a year, working at least twenty-four hours a week, and that your annual income is equal to or greater than the cost of health insurance premiums. So even if you have a preexisting condition like bipolar disorder, your babysitting business or freelance writing could qualify you for group health insurance.

ASSOCIATIONS

Some alumni associations, trade organizations, and chambers of commerce offer group coverage health insurance to their members. (Guys, it's never too late to become a Freemason. Never. Too. Late.) But do your research. The plans offered by alumni associations and other organizations can only help you if they're not medically underwritten (i.e., if they can't deny you based on preexisting conditions). Even organizations like the Writer's Union offer health insurance in some states. Check it out.

STATE-SPONSORED HIGH-RISK POOLS

Most states have high-risk insurance pools you can buy into. They were specifically created for people like us, who can't get insurance by any other means. These pools are often expensive, but it's better than having no insurance at all. You can find information about your state's high-risk pool by searching "[state name] high risk pool" on the Web. These plans run $300 to $400 a month, so let's hope your parents are paying for it.

PART 4: BOTTOM-OF-THE-BARREL OPTIONS FOR GETTING INSURED

GET HITCHED

If your significant other has a job that provides health insurance, you can always marry him/her and get on his/

her health insurance as a dependent. Employers are legally required to let their employees' uninsured spouses onto the health plan without a waiting period. Boo-ya, here comes the bride!

MEDICAID

You might be eligible for Medicaid, the federally funded, state-administered health program for low-income and disabled people. Eligibility requirements vary by state, but in general you qualify if you're on SSI/SSP (see below), are pregnant, have a child, or are blind, over sixty-five, or disabled. Check out your state eligibility requirements. It can't hurt to apply if you think you're eligible: the worst they can do is decline you, and you just might get in.

SSI

If you want to get Medicaid, you need to be on SSI (Supplemental Security Income). To qualify for SSI, you must be old, blind, or disabled *and* have limited income and resources.

Let's break it down.

Having bipolar disorder doesn't automatically make you disabled. Your bipolar disorder only qualifies as a disability if it's so severe that you're unable to support yourself by holding down a steady job. The DDS (Disability Determination Service) only considers you disabled if you're unable to perform "substantial gainful activity" that is, unable to do productive, useful things that normally make money. The DDS really gets into it: if you're capable of basic tasks like raking leaves five days a week or hanging out in a Smokey the Bear costume, you might get turned down for SSI. They look at both physical and mental abilities. Even if you're completely healthy physically, you can still qualify for SSI if your bipolar disorder has rendered you incapable of earning enough dough to pay for food and rent.

The DDS determines how crazy you are by looking at your medical records. Therefore, if you haven't been seeing a psychiatrist regularly and don't have a history of being institutionalized, they won't have much to look at, and it will be hard to convince them you're truly needy. And if you're not truly needy, you shouldn't be applying for SSI.

If the DDS accepts that you're batshit crazy (at least on paper) and can't make enough to support yourself, you also need to prove you're poor.

How poor?

It varies by state, but generally, you have to be making less than $700 to $900 a month and own less than $2,000 worth of "resources" (e.g., land, cash, bank accounts, stuff you could sell to buy food or pay rent). The state will hunt down all your financial records to make sure you're not lying about how much money you have.

If you get accepted for SSI, the state will pay you a certain amount of money each month. How much you get is determined by a few factors, namely your living situation and income. The more income you have, whether in the form of gifts or money earned from a job, the less money SSI will give you. Also, you get more money if you're paying rent than if you're living rent-free with your uncle or boyfriend/girlfriend. Currently, the maximum monthly SSI payment is about $640.

SSI is hard to get and easy to lose. There are lots of rules. You can't leave the country, get a well-paying job, or even live anywhere you want to live and still get benefits. You should apply only if you're really incapable of supporting yourself. If you just apply because you think bipolar disorder is a get-out-of-work-free card, you're a jackass and will probably be declined.

Either way, if you play the SSI game, be ready for some headaches. Big Brother is so-o-o watching.

GET KNOCKED UP

You automatically qualify for Medicaid if you're preggo and poor. Just saying.

BLIND YOURSELF

You automatically qualify for Medicaid if you're blind and poor. Just saying.

GET KNOCKED UP AND BLIND YOURSELF

Twice the eligibility, yo!

RICH UNCLE/RICH GREAT-AUNT/ CORPORATE SPONSOR/ANONYMOUS SPONSOR

OK, here's a crazy idea. What if there was a website that matched cute, adorable, uninsurable bipolar twenty-somethings with wealthy corporate or private sponsors who would sign up to pay said twenty-something's expensive high-risk pool health insurance premiums? The recipient could send the donor smiley photographs and cheerful handwritten letters from time to time, and the donor would have the pleasure of knowing they were keeping a fine upstanding young person stocked with lithium and therapy so said young person grows up big and strong and doesn't end up living in a bathroom stall at the library (e.g., spaceship command center ZX7182). Um, someone with web skills want to get on this?

PRESCRIPTION ASSISTANCE

Did you know that most pharmaceutical companies offer discounts and/or financial aid to people without insurance? Bonanza! I looked into it, and there's a program for pretty much any brand or generic drug you might be taking for bipolar. You have to be a U.S. resident, uninsured, and making less than a certain amount of money per year—usually around $30,000. Once you're approved, the company sends a three-month supply of your drug to your doctor. You need to contact the program for refills and reapply once a year.

BECOME A CANADIAN

Or a Brit. Or a German. Or a citizen of some other country with universal health care. I'm a dual citizen of the United States and Canada, and when I lived in Vancouver, I could go to a walk-in clinic, spend fifteen minutes in the waiting room, see a doctor, and pay nothing for it. Since moving to the United States, I've been appalled at the injustice of the health-care system—from being denied coverage for having a mental illness to being charged hundreds of dollars for the privilege of seeing a doctor for eight and a half minutes to get a prescription. This country's health-care system is evil and insane. And writing about it is making me really edgy, so

I'm going to end this paragraph right now and move o
to something else.

PART 5: EVERYTHING YOU KNOW IS WRONG
OR ABOUT TO CHANGE

All of the above might be about to change. Maybe. As
you might be aware, we swore in a new president in
2009, and he promised massive reforms to the U.S.
health-care system. If these reforms go through, we
could be looking at a whole new system, a system in
which anyone—yes, even you—can get reasonably
priced health insurance, regardless of preexisting medical conditions. Under this new system, you could be
bleeding out the eyeballs, and you'd still qualify for any
health plan you wanted, at the same price as everyone else. Now's the time to get our act together and
rally for these changes, to make sure they go through.
Obama promised universal health care in his first term.
A first term lasts four years. Imagine being done with
asshole insurance companies, exorbitant "bipolar" insurance rates, and similar discrimination in four short
years. Wonderful, if it actually happens.

Let's have a little taste of the goods. The points of
Obama's health plan that are of most interest to mental-
health consumers are:

- *Guaranteed eligibility*
  Under Obama's plan, all health insurance companies across
  America would have to extend guaranteed eligibility to all
  Americans, regardless of preexisting conditions, at "fair and

stable premiums." This means health insurance companies could no longer deny you or charge you exorbitant rates because you have bipolar disorder or another mental illness.

- *Raising age of dependence to twenty-five*
  Obama wants all states to do what some have already done: raise the age of health insurance dependence. This means you'd be able to stay on your parents' plan as a "dependent" until you were twenty-five, instead of getting kicked off sooner. Makes sense to me.

- *More options for drugs*
  Under Obama's plan, Americans would finally be allowed to buy prescription drugs from developed countries like Canada. Due to a variety of screwed-up laws, this would actually be cheaper than buying them in the United States. Obama also wants to push through legislation that would stop drug companies from blocking consumer access to generics. In short: cheaper drugs for all.

As of this writing, nobody knows which of these reforms will actually go through. There's been a lot of opposition from conservative organizations and from health insurance companies who are afraid of losing their profits. Plus, Obama hasn't given a timetable for his proposed reforms or mentioned if the changes would be incremental or part of a comprehensive package.

Regardless, being treated like a second-class citizen is getting mighty tiring. Change, anyone?

CONCLUSION

Quick!

Life is a video game. At birth everyone is given the same set of controllers: you can run, jump, duck, or shoot. For a long time, it seems like everyone is playing the same game. You hear other people's beeps and boops and power-up noises all around. You do your best to collect all the treasures and bonk the bad guys on the head, and assume everyone else is doing the same.

Then one day you discover everyone is *not* playing the same game: some people's game involves lots of gold coins, some people are stuck in the Crystal Castle looking for love, some people are sloshing through an underwater level you've never even seen before.

And you—your game is faster and harder than the others. The rules keep changing. One minute you need to bang on the jump button ten times per second just to keep your character from drowning, and the next you're battling the Big Boss in an antigravity chamber a thousand years in the future. You're down to half a heart, then up to full hearts plus a bonus one. If you don't collect enough mushrooms, the scenery starts to change and the music gets weird.

You start to get mad because your game is so hard. You keep having to start over again each time something goes wrong. Sometimes you're not sure you even care if your little character lives or dies.

Hold up.

You, like everyone else in the world, have exactly four options available to you. You can run, jump, duck, or shoot. You can't control the monsters and bosses that are coming at you, but with a little practice you can develop your own unique strategy, philosophy, and game wisdom for making it through the round. You *care* about your little guy and talk him through tough situations. You develop thumbs the size of baguettes from handling the controller, and an aura of wise unflappability other gamers envy and admire.

———◆———

This is not a book to tell you exactly what bipolar disorder is or how not to have it anymore. This book is just a way of saying, "Hey, you and me and a million other people have a few things in common. Here are some ways of thinking about it, and some ways of helping ourselves through it." Bipolar—or whatever you want to call it—is for life, and the sooner we wrestle mental illness out of the realm of stigma and discrimination and into the realm of "Hey—I'm a whole person, whose game happens to include manic and depressive monster bosses," the faster the world will become a safer, happier place for ourselves and people like us.

So take what you like from this book and leave the rest. Find your own metaphors for bipolar—whatever helps you understand your experience and express it to other people.

Live large. Think big. Go for walks.

See you on the flip side.

Hilary

RESOURCES

ACTIVE MINDS

www.activeminds.org

Active Minds is a student mental-health organization with chapters on over two hundred college and university campuses. Active Minds chapters offer support and advocacy for students with mental illnesses and these students' allies, and they organize events like speakers and mental-health movie nights.

DEPRESSION AND BIPOLAR SUPPORT ALLIANCE (DBSA)

www.dbsalliance.org

The DBSA is a mental-health organization with a focus on education, advocacy, and peer support. It runs mental-health training seminars for the friends and family of people with mental illnesses, sponsor over a thousand patient-run support groups (find one near you!), and publish tons of free educational materials about bipolar, depression, and schizophrenia.

THE ICARUS PROJECT

www.theicarusproject.net

The Icarus Project is the biggest, most well-organized mad pride organization you can find on the Internet. Its mantra is "navigating the space between brilliance and madness." Its website has articles, forums, and community resources for mental health.

NATIONAL ALLIANCE FOR MENTAL ILLNESS (NAMI)

www.nami.org

NAMI is the biggest mental-health organization in, like, the world. Its website is ground zero for news, information, community resources, and forums on all things mental illness. It's also a good place to get involved in mental-health advocacy, from letter-writing campaigns to protests.

CRAZYMEDS

www.crazymeds.us

Crazymeds is the place to go for exhaustive information on the meds you're taking. The site is run by Jerod Poore, a "citizen medical expert" who himself has autism and bipolar disorder. In addition to regularly updated drug info, there are message boards where you can connect with other people who take crazy meds.

HALF OF US

www.halfofus.com

Half of Us is a big-budget, college mental-health awareness campaign with a pretty great website. The site features videos and stories from youth with mental illnesses and information on subjects that are too often silent on college campuses, including suicide, self-injury, and drug abuse.

NATIONAL INSTITUTE OF MENTAL HEALTH (NIMH)
www.nimh.nih.gov

NIMH is a government-funded organization that publishes news and research on mental-health topics. It's a good place to read about the latest clinical trials or the results of studies about bipolar, schizophrenia, and depression. Keep it in mind for your next research paper.

GOOD NONFICTION BOOKS ABOUT BIPOLAR AND DEPRESSION

Antonetta, Suzanne. *A Mind Apart: Travels in a Neurodiverse World*. New York: Tarcher, 2005.

Castle, Lana. *Finding Your Bipolar Muse: How to Master Depressive Droughts and Manic Floods and Access Your Creative Power*. New York: Marlow & Company, 2006.

Gardner, John. *The Hypomanic Edge: The Link Between (A Little) Craziness and (A Lot) of Success in America*. New York: Simon and Schuster, 2005.

Jamison, Kay Redfield. *An Unquiet Mind: A Memoir of Moods and Madness*. New York: Vintage Books, 1996.

————. *Touched with Fire: Manic-Depressive Illness and the Creative Temperament*. New York: The Free Press, 1993.

NATIONAL CRISIS HOTLINES

NATIONAL SUICIDE PREVENTION LIFELINE

1-800-273-TALK

National 24/7 suicide crisis hotline. Call for free from any phone, any time, to speak with a trained counselor. Your call will be routed to the closest crisis center in your area, and whoever you talk to will be able to direct you to further help once the call is over. Also available in Spanish.

NATIONAL RUNAWAY SWITCHBOARD

1-800-RUNAWAY

If you're between the ages of twelve and twenty and have run away from home (for example, during a manic episode), you can call this number to arrange a free Greyhound ride back to your folks. The switchboard operators will also connect you with resources and counseling if your family is having conflicts.

ABOUT THE AUTHOR

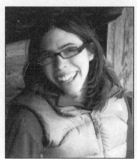

Photograph © Gabriel Jacobs

Hilary Smith studied English Literature at the University of British Columbia, where she was diagnosed with bipolar disorder after one too many insomniac bike rides in her junior year. She is the editor of *The Med Magazine,* an online satire magazine for young people with mental illnesses *(www.themedmagazine.com)* and writes for suite101 *(www.suite101.com).* Hilary lives in the Pacific Northwest and is working on her first young adult novel.

TO OUR READERS

Conari Press, an imprint of Red Wheel/Weiser, publishes books on topics ranging from spirituality, personal growth, and relationships to women's issues, parenting, and social issues. Our mission is to publish quality books that will make a difference in people's lives—how we feel about ourselves and how we relate to one another. We value integrity, compassion, and receptivity, both in the books we publish and in the way we do business.

Our readers are our most important resources, and we value your input, suggestions, and ideas about what you would like to see published. Please feel free to contact us, to request our latest book catalog, or to be added to our mailing list.

Conari Press
An imprint of Red Wheel/Weiser, LLC
500 Third Street, Suite 230
San Francisco, CA 94107
www.redwheelweiser.com